Psychodynamic Treatment of Depression

SECOND EDITION

Fredric N. Busch, M.D.
Clinical Professor of Psychiatry,
Weill Medical College of Cornell University
Faculty, Columbia University Center for
Psychoanalytic Training and Research
New York, New York

Marie Rudden, M.D.
Clinical Assistant Professor of Psychiatry,
Weill Medical College of Cornell University
New York, New York; Training and Supervising Analyst,
Berkshire Psychoanalytic Institute

Theodore Shapiro, M.D.
Emeritus Professor of Psychiatry in Pediatrics,
Weill Medical College of Cornell University
Training and Supervising Analyst,
New York Psychoanalytic Institute
New York, New York

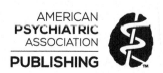

AMERICAN
PSYCHIATRIC
ASSOCIATION
PUBLISHING

D1518143

If you wish to buy 50 or more copies of the same title, please go to www.appi.org/special discounts for more information.

Copyright © 2016 American Psychiatric Association
ALL RIGHTS RESERVED

Manufactured in the United States of America on acid-free paper
20 19 18 17 16   5 4 3 2 1
Second Edition

Typeset in Adobe's AGaramond and Formata

American Psychiatric Publishing, Inc.
1000 Wilson Boulevard
Arlington, VA 22209-3901
www.appi.org

Library of Congress Cataloging-in-Publication Data
Names: Busch, Fredric, author. | Rudden, Marie, author. | Shapiro, Theodore, author. | American Psychiatric Association, issuing body.
Title: Psychodynamic treatment of depression / by Fredric N. Busch, Marie Rudden, Theodore Shapiro.
Description: Second edition. | Arlington, Virginia : American Psychiatric Association Publishing, [2016] | Includes bibliographical references and index.
Identifiers: LCCN 2016000271 (print) | LCCN 2016000908 (ebook) | ISBN 9781615370351 (pbk. : alk. paper) | ISBN 9781615370696 ()
Subjects: | MESH: Depressive Disorder—therapy | Personality Disorders—therapy | Psychotherapy, Psychodynamic—methods | Case Reports
Classification: LCC RC537 (print) | LCC RC537 (ebook) | NLM WM 171.5 | DDC 616.85/270651—dc23
LC record available at http://lccn.loc.gov/2016000271

British Library Cataloguing in Publication Data
A CIP record is available from the British Library.

Psychodynamic Treatment of Depression

SECOND EDITION

Contents

PART III
Special Topics

PART I

Introduction and Overview

Introduction

The Value and Limitations of Current Treatment Approaches to Depressive Disorders

There has been remarkable progress in the treatment of depression. Multiple effective psychopharmacological interventions and psychotherapeutic treatments are in current use. Cognitive-behavioral therapy, interpersonal psychotherapy, and psychopharmacological treatments have all been demonstrated, in placebo-controlled studies, to be effective in treating major depression (e.g., see the review of treatment studies in American Psychiatric Association 2010).

Clinicians are aware, however, that treatment of depression often continues to be a struggle. Many patients' depression does not respond fully to these interventions, and some patients have persistent social and occupational deficits (American Psychiatric Association 2010). There is a significant rate of recurrence of major depressive disorder (Eaton et al. 2008). Chronic depression with prolonged episodes and persistent symptoms between episodes is common (Judd et al. 1997; Keller et al. 1996; Kocsis and Klein 1995) and shows lower response rates than nonchronic depression (American Psychiatric Association 2010). Continuous subsyndromal symptoms or symptoms of "minor" depression can cause functional impairment and persistent suffering (Rapaport et al. 2002; Vieta et al. 2008). Therefore, there is increasing emphasis on the importance of patients' recovery from depression (a return to baseline functioning) rather than response to treatment (at least a 50% reduction of symptoms), which is usually used as the criterion in treatment studies for determining effectiveness (Keller 2003; Thase 1999). It is important, then, to develop treatments or combinations of treatments that address more fully the neurophysiological and psychological vulnerabilities that may predispose patients to persistent symptoms or recurrences of depression. Psychotherapeutic treatment of depression may aid in the prevention of relapse, and psychodynamic psychotherapy should be considered and investigated as an approach to reducing this vulnerability (Gabbard et al. 2002).

Clinicians tend to use combined approaches and attempt to determine the most effective combinations of treatment for individual patients, and evidence suggests an advantage of combined over single treatment in some cases (Busch and Sandberg 2012). However, the presence of persistent and troubling side effects from antidepressant medication often leads to a search for alternative antidepressant or psychotherapeutic interventions. Just as patients' responses to medications vary, responses to particular therapeutic interventions are different in different patients. Psychodynamic psychotherapy explores internal conflicts and unconscious issues that are often not addressed in cognitive-behavioral, interpersonal, or medication treatments.

The Evidence Base for Psychodynamic Approaches to Depressive Disorders

Increasingly, studies of psychodynamic psychotherapy have demonstrated effectiveness in randomized controlled trials (Driessen et al. 2010; Leichsenring et al. 2015). Although there are concerns about the quality of these studies (Abbass et al. 2014), these problems are also present in studies of other psychotherapies, and studies have been improving in quality over time (Thoma et al. 2012). Burnand et al. (2002) compared psychodynamic psychotherapy plus clomipramine with clomipramine alone in a randomized, controlled trial in patients with major depression. Combined treatment was more cost-effective, and the combined-treatment group showed fewer treatment failures and better functioning. Driessen et al. (2010) found that psychodynamic psychotherapy was comparable to cognitive-behavioral therapy in a large randomized controlled trial. From this study, Thase (2013) concluded: "On the basis of these findings, there is no reason to believe that psychodynamic psychotherapy is a less effective treatment of major depressive disorder than CBT [cognitive-behavioral therapy]" (p. 954).

Despite increasing evidence regarding psychodynamic psychotherapy in the treatment of depression, it is still limited relative to other psychotherapies. *Practice Guideline for the Treatment of Patients With Major Depressive Disorder*, 3rd Edition (American Psychiatric Association 2010) recommends additional, more rigorously designed studies of psychodynamic psychotherapeutic treatment of depression. In addition, more studies need to be done assessing the impact of various treatments on long-term vulnerability to persistent symptoms and recurrence and in selected populations.

Indications for Psychodynamic Treatment of Depression

The psychodynamic approach presented in this book is adapted and molded to address the specific dynamisms that we have found to drive depressive symptoms and syndromes. The therapy outlined is applicable to the internal struggles that contribute to affective disorders and that are complementary to the biological source of some depressive illnesses. We therefore suggest that focused psychodynamic psychotherapy can be a valuable adjunct for the treatment of depression, including the vulnerability to recurrence of depression, and that in some cases it may be effective alone.

Because the dynamics of depression involving narcissistic vulnerability, self-directed rage, shame, and guilt are explored with this method and are carefully delineated with patients, it is likely that this treatment is helpful for a range of depressive disorders and subclinical depressive syndromes. In the absence of systematic research, however, we cannot make any definitive statement about the specificity of these dynamics or the effectiveness of this approach in all depressive disorders. On the basis of clinical experience, we recommend this approach primarily in patients with mild or moderate major depression and chronic persistent depression (dysthymia) as per DSM-5 (American Psychiatric Association 2013). However, we do suggest that patients with bipolar disorder and more severe major depressive disorders also may be aided by psychodynamic psychotherapy when their symptoms are adequately controlled with medication. Affective or ideational contents of depression are most likely to respond to this treatment, although vegetative symptoms sometimes respond as well. Issues of combining psychodynamic psychotherapy with medication or other adjunctive treatments are discussed below and in Chapter 15 ("Use of Psychodynamic Psychotherapy With Other Treatment Approaches") in this volume.

In addition, from clinical experience, we believe this approach may be of particular value in treatment of patients with depressive disorders and comorbid personality disorders. Comorbid personality disorders have been found to have an adverse effect on treatment outcome (Corruble et al. 1996; Friborg et al. 2014), including diminished response to antidepressants, reduced adherence to treatment, and longer time period to achieve remission (American Psychiatric Association 2010). The rate of comorbidity between these disorders is high: 37.9% in one major epidemiological study (Hasin et al. 2005). We have therefore added a chapter in this edition on approaches to some personality disorders found to be comorbid with depressive disorders (see Chapter 12, "Psychodynamic Approaches to Depression With Comorbid Personality Disorder").

This book, then, offers a psychotherapeutic approach to the dynamics observed in depressed patients that can sharpen clinicians' treatment skills. We present many clinical case vignettes to illustrate common dynamic constellations and techniques for engaging patients in depression-focused psychodynamic psychotherapy. Through the vignettes, we attempt to capture the essence of clinical work with such patients rather than present a verbatim record of our sessions, but all are quite closely based on material from therapy with depressed patients in our practices or in supervision. These vignettes highlight effective therapeutic interventions. It should be noted, however, that many cases have periods in which therapy is frustrating and difficult, interventions seem unhelpful, and the therapist struggles for ways to resolve the impasse. Dealing with more complex and frustrating cases of depression is addressed in Chapter 13 ("Managing Impasses and Negative Reactions to Treatment") in this volume. Some details have been altered in these case presentations to protect our patients' confidentiality, but the dynamic issues remain true to the clinical data.

Background Training

Our intention is that this book be used by clinicians who are trained in the practice of psychotherapy and in the diagnosis of depression and related character disorders. We recommend that supervision by psychoanalysts or by dynamically trained therapists be sought by those practitioners who are not themselves trained in psychodynamic techniques. It takes some experience to recognize the dynamics that we describe here, as well as to identify and work with the transference and countertransference paradigms seen frequently in depressed patients and described in detail in Chapter 5 ("The Middle Phase of Treatment") in this volume.

Initial Evaluation and Determining the Appropriateness of Psychodynamic Psychotherapy

The initial evaluation of the depressed patient should include both an assessment of depressive symptoms and of the patient's capacity to benefit from psychodynamic treatment. The clinician reviews the patient's developmental history, relationships, stressors, and conflicts. The clinician employs a semistructured interview and should follow up on topics that trigger a depressed mood or defensiveness. At all times, the clinician is sensitive to linkages, word usage, repetitions, and omissions that stamp the delivery of the narrative. Important topics to explore in the evaluation are summarized in Table 1–1.

Several patient characteristics are felt to be conducive to psychodynamic treatment, such as 1) a motivation to understand the sources of symptoms, 2) the ability to think psychologically, 3) the capacity to have and think about meaningful and complex relationships with others, 4) the capacity for control over impulses, 5) the ability to understand metaphors, 6) the capacity to acknowledge emotional states, and 7) good reality testing. In the course of the initial interviews, the therapist should observe the patient's ability to understand and respond to probes about the meaning of the symptoms and preliminary interpretations regarding the source of the symptoms. Relative contraindications include 1) marked difficulty observing the self or reflecting on others' motivations, 2) significant inability to tolerate frustration, 3) globally impaired relationships, 4) marked difficulty forming an alliance with the therapist, 5) low intelligence, and 6) a severe depression that disrupts the patient's ability to work effectively in psychotherapy.

Although these characteristics are of value, patients without these characteristics can respond to psychodynamic treatment (Busch et al. 1999). A broader array of patients can work effectively in a more structured psychodynamic treatment that focuses on specific symptoms and their associated dynamics. Many patients can be taught the psychodynamic approach, such as learning to observe internal emotions and motivations more closely and considering that symptoms may have unconscious sources. In those instances

---

Table 1–1.   Important topics to explore in the initial evaluation of the depressed patient

---

Assessment of depression

- Depressive symptoms as delineated in DSM-5 (American Psychiatric Association 2013) as well as unique or idiosyncratic descriptions of symptoms
- Stressors, circumstances, and feelings that preceded the onset of depression
- Prior depressive episodes and the circumstances surrounding them, such as precipitating events and stressors, with a focus on eliciting accompanying feelings and fantasies

Developmental and family history

- Family management of emotions in the patient's childhood and adolescence, including sadness, depression, shame, anger, and anxiety, particularly with regard to losses, illnesses, or separations
- Childhood depressive symptoms
- Perceptions of parental attitudes and behaviors
- Adult relationships: characteristics and qualities of relationships, including conflicts, emotional themes, and perceived level of responsiveness of significant others
- Family history of depressive disorders; family attitudes toward this history

Assessment of the patient's capacities to work in an exploratory psychodynamic psychotherapy

- Ability to describe feelings, fantasies, and interpersonal relationships
- Presence of curiosity about the emotional origins of the symptoms
- Ability to respond to a trial linkage and/or interpretation with reflection, curiosity, or new associations

---

in which these capacities are more limited or absent, the clinician would initially include more psychoeducational interventions.

The following cases illustrate one instance in which psychological mindedness was present but was inhibited and another in which the patient's limited psychological capacity interfered with his ability to work effectively in a psychodynamic treatment.

Case Example 1

Mr. A, a prominent lawyer in his 40s, was quite reluctant to seek treatment for depression that had gradually escalated over the course of many months. He seemed ashamed to admit to any vulnerability and initially had difficulty engaging in a psychodynamic treatment. It became increasingly apparent to his therapist, over the course of their initial consultation, that Mr. A had a tendency to take on herculean tasks and to relentlessly push himself to accomplish them. This seemed to have started when his parents were divorced and he had taken on, as an adolescent, a major portion of responsibility for the family business. He had usually been quite successful at these endeavors and was widely admired, but he had recently accepted a task that, for dynamic reasons requiring further exploration, he could not allow himself to accomplish. The shame and guilt that resulted from this failure were crippling him now and interfering with his ability to openly explore the origins of his symptoms.

When his therapist outlined this very cursory early understanding of her patient, Mr. A began to sob. "No one ever listens the way you just did," he murmured. "Maybe I don't let them; maybe I signal them that that's not okay. But no one has listened so carefully since a close friend of mine died."

Mr. A's thwarted longings for understanding became a powerful motivating force in his treatment. As it unfolded, his desire to be understood by others sometimes eclipsed his wish to actively understand himself, but this became part of the work of the therapy at a later phase. Once his shame and fears of vulnerability began to be addressed, Mr. A evidenced an ability to reflect about himself and his impact on others. His comment "Maybe I don't let them…" was a valuable indicator that he could look at himself in relation to others and consider the impact of his own behavior on their responses. Other patients need to be encouraged to consider this viewpoint and can steadily develop this capacity.

Case Example 2

Mr. B seemed, from the initial interviews, to need his therapist's understanding and help in a very concrete manner. A college professor in his 30s, Mr. B implored her to respond to his frequent phone calls and complained bitterly about the frustrations he had experienced in previous therapies. The experience of attachment and connection in the therapeutic engagement, and of having an audience to witness his reported unjust treatment at the hands of his parents and coworkers, seemed paramount to him, even as, sadly, he despised himself for needing and wanting this support. He presented with a concrete appraisal of the origins of his depression and seemed unable to be curious about himself in any other light. He found it extremely difficult to evaluate his impact on others, despite many attempts by his therapist to encourage this kind of reflection in their early sessions. For instance, he interpreted her fairly mild questions about why a coworker might be angry with him (something that seemed quite obvious to his therapist from a brief description of their quarrel) in a paranoid way, insisting that she was unsympathetic and oddly hostile.

The motivation that seemed to consume Mr. B above all was his need to describe his suffering at the hands of others and to seek almost magical relief from his pain about this. Although this may be an aspect of the treatment motivation of some depressed patients, it must be accompanied by a desire to understand the other's injurious behavior and to consider the possibility that the patient may be provoking this behavior out of his own awareness, in order for an exploratory treatment to hold much promise.

After a yearlong treatment that was deeply frustrating at times for both therapist and patient, Mr. B acknowledged begrudgingly that he had learned a good deal about himself, but he said that at that point he wished to pursue a more practical treatment. His therapist concurred that their effort had produced results, notably a greater capacity for empathy, a diminishment of his rigidly paranoid stance, and a somewhat reduced tendency to self-hatred, and agreed to refer him for behavioral treatment, as Mr. B remained reluctant to explore his tendency to depression further.

Thus, the clinician should be aware that some patients, because of limitations in their reflective capacities, find it quite difficult to work in an insight-oriented psychotherapy and should be flexible when considering alternate treatment interventions.

Length of Treatment

Psychodynamic treatment of depression can be employed either as a brief psychotherapy (approximately 3–6 months) aimed at relief of depressive symptoms or as a longer-term treatment (approximately 6 months to 2 years) aimed at reduction of characterological and intrapsychic vulnerabilities to recurrence of depression. Some patients with recurrent depression, chronic persistent depression (dysthymia), and entrenched character pathology (e.g., borderline personality disorder), however, may require more than 2 years of treatment. Although a short-term treatment can aid in developing some understanding of the conflicts that trigger depressive symptoms, therapists and patients often recognize that a more lengthy treatment may be needed to comprehend more fully those personality problems, internal conflicts, and problematic relationships that can increase the patient's vulnerability to depression. In addition, because conflicts are frequently unconscious, a longer-term treatment can provide an opportunity to ascertain more clearly factors that operate out of the patient's awareness. Once these factors are understood, psychotherapy can help the patient to modify them.

Recommending Psychodynamic Treatment of Depression and Possible Adjunctive Use of Medication

Once the clinician recommends psychodynamic psychotherapy to the patient, the patient should be informed of the risks and benefits of the various interventions used for depression, in order to take part in the decision-making process. One important consideration is whether medications should be used in conjunction with a psychodynamic treatment. Factors to consider include the severity of depressive symptoms and the level of disruption in concentration and motivation. For a fuller discussion of these issues, see Chapter 15.

Patients frequently struggle to understand how a combination of treatments can be helpful for their symptoms. They may be interested in learning why such disparate interventions as psychotherapy and medications may be effective, or they may be unwilling to employ a combination of treatments because they are unsure how both could be helpful. Although not physiologically accurate, certain metaphors may be of value in aiding the patient's understanding of the use of complementary interventions.

One helpful model uses hypertension as an analogue for depression. Stress, poor diet, overweight, and physiological propensities can all contribute to hypertension. Changes in the first of those three characteristics can lead to decreases in blood pressure and may obviate the need for medication. However, in some patients these interventions would be inadequate. If blood pressure is too high, it is more imminently dangerous, and medication should be given even while other changes are employed.

In using this analogy with the patient, the therapist can describe psychotherapy for depression as equivalent to stress reduction and dietary changes. As with hypertension, in some patients the depression may respond to these interventions, whereas in other individuals medication may be needed. In some cases, the depression may be highly disruptive to functioning or even dangerous, requiring medication more immediately.

A diathesis model may also enhance understanding, suggesting that the patient has a biological propensity for depressive disorders. Psychodynamic models can aid in identifying what intrapsychic and interpersonal factors may trigger this tendency.

Overview of This Book

In the chapters that immediately follow, we offer a historical review of the literature leading up to our working dynamic formulation for depressive disorders, along with an overview of the treatment.

The middle section of this book focuses on the techniques of psychodynamic psychotherapy as they particularly apply to treating patients with depression. Individual chapters highlight techniques to help patients recognize their vulnerability to the dynamics that form the core of the depressive experience and illustrate how to work with these techniques to help patients better manage their vulnerability.

Finally, we address certain topics of special concern in the psychotherapy of depression. Chapter 12 ("Psychodynamic Approaches to Depression With Comorbid Personality Disorder") focuses on the comorbidity of personality disorders and depressive disorders. Chapter 13 ("Managing Impasses and Negative Reactions to Treatment") discusses approaches for addressing complex cases and treatment impasses. Chapter 14 ("Psychodynamic Approaches to Suicidality") offers a psychodynamic perspective on helping patients to better understand and manage their suicidal thoughts and impulses. Finally, issues to consider when combining treatments are discussed in Chapter 15.

References

Abbass AA, Kisely SR, Town JM, et al: Short-term psychodynamic psychotherapies for common mental disorders. Cochrane Database Syst Rev 7:CD004687, 2014 24984083

American Psychiatric Association: Practice guideline for the treatment of patients with major depressive disorder (Third Edition). Am J Psychiatry 157(suppl):1–45, 2010

American Psychiatric Association: Diagnostic and Statistical Manual of Mental Disorders, 5th Edition. Arlington, VA, American Psychiatric Association, 2013

Burnand Y, Andreoli A, Kolatte E, et al: Psychodynamic psychotherapy and clomipramine in the treatment of major depression. Psychiatr Serv 53:585–590, 2002

Busch FN, Sandberg LS: Combined treatment of depression. Psychiatr Clin North Am 35(1):165–179, 2012 22370497

Busch FN, Milrod BL, Singer MB: Theory and technique in psychodynamic treatment of panic disorder. J Psychother Pract Res 8(3):234–242, 1999 10413443

Corruble E, Ginestet D, Guelfi JD: Comorbidity of personality disorders and unipolar major depression: a review. J Affect Disord 37(2-3):157–170, 1996 8731079

Driessen E, Cuijpers P, de Maat SC, et al: The efficacy of short-term psychodynamic psychotherapy for depression: a meta-analysis. Clin Psych Rev 30(1):25–36, 2010 19766369

Eaton WW, Shao H, Nestadt G, et al: Population-based study of first onset and chronicity in major depressive disorder. Arch Gen Psychiatry 65(5):513–520, 2008 18458203

Friborg O, Martinsen EW, Martinussen M, et al: Comorbidity of personality disorders in mood disorders: a meta-analytic review of 122 studies from 1988 to 2010. J Affect Disord 152-154:1–11, 2014 24120406

Gabbard GO, Gunderson JG, Fonagy P: The place of psychoanalytic treatments within psychiatry. Arch Gen Psychiatry 59(6):505–510, 2002 12044192

Hasin DS, Goodwin RD, Stinson FS, Grant BF: Epidemiology of major depressive disorder: results from the National Epidemiologic Survey on Alcoholism and Related Conditions. Arch Gen Psychiatry 62(10):1097–1106, 2005 16203955

Judd LL, Akiskal HS, Paulus MP: The role and clinical significance of subsyndromal depressive symptoms (SSD) in unipolar major depressive disorder. J Affect Disord 45(1-2):5–17, discussion 17–18, 1997 9268771

Keller MB: Past, present, and future directions for defining optimal treatment outcome in depression: remission and beyond. JAMA 289(23):3152–3160, 2003 12813121

Keller MB, Hanks DL, Klein DN: Summary of the DSM-IV mood disorders field trial and issue overview. Psychiatr Clin North Am 19(1):1–28, 1996 8677213

Kocsis JH, Klein DN (eds): Diagnosis and Treatment of Chronic Depression. New York, Guilford, 1995

Leichsenring F, Leweke F, Klein S, Steinert C: The empirical status of psychodynamic psychotherapy—an update: Bambi's alive and kicking. Psychother Psychosom 84(3):129–148, 2015 25833321

Rapaport MH, Judd LL, Schettler PJ, et al: A descriptive analysis of minor depression. Am J Psychiatry 159(4):637–643, 2002 11925303

Thase ME: Redefining antidepressant efficacy toward long-term recovery. J Clin Psychiatry 60 (suppl 6):15–19, 1999 10235120

Thase ME: Comparative effectiveness of psychodynamic psychotherapy and cognitive-behavioral therapy: it's about time, and what's next? Am J Psychiatry 170(9):953–956, 2013 24030607

Thoma NC, McKay D, Gerber AJ, et al: A quality-based review of randomized controlled trials of cognitive-behavioral therapy for depression: an assessment and metaregression. Am J Psychiatry 169(1):22–30, 2012 22193528

Vieta E, Sánchez-Moreno J, Lahuerta J, Zaragoza S; EDHIPO Group (Hypomania Detection Study Group): Subsyndromal depressive symptoms in patients with bipolar and unipolar disorder during clinical remission. J Affect Disord 107(1-3):169–174, 2008 17870184

Development of a Psychodynamic Model of Depression

THEORISTS have developed a variety of models to explain why certain individuals develop depressive disorders and to aid in the planning of treatment. Vulnerability to depression has been explained variously in terms of biochemical, interpersonal, and cognitive-behavioral models. Other theorists have used a psychodynamic model to explain the complex set of feelings and behaviors that make up depressive disorders. This book focuses on the psychodynamic approach as a comprehensive means of understanding and treating depression that is complementary to the other models and approaches. In this chapter we provide a brief summary of psychoanalytic theories of depression, describe studies of psychological contributions to the disorder, and present a psychodynamic formulation that can be employed in guiding treatment.

Psychoanalysts have developed successive, overlapping models to explain the etiology and persistence of depressive syndromes. These models have considered the individual's biological and temperamental vulnerabilities, the quality of the person's earliest attachment relationships, and significant childhood experiences that may have been accompanied by frustration, shame, loss, helplessness, loneliness, or guilt. The impact of such experiences and feelings during formative developmental stages on individuals' perceptions of themselves and others is seen as creating dynamic susceptibilities to a range of depressive syndromes later in life, including narcissistic vulnerability, conflicted anger, excessively high expectations of self and others, and maladaptive defense mechanisms.

To best illustrate the various psychodynamic models of depression, we describe their application to a specific case.

Case Example

Ms. C was an overweight, 45-year-old divorced accountant who presented for treatment with a history of several years of dysthymic symptoms and multiple episodes of superimposed major depression. During depressive episodes, her symptoms included very low energy and motivation, impaired concentration, increased appetite with weight gain, and middle and terminal insomnia. Ms. C viewed herself as worthless and not deserving of attention from other people at the same time that she was furious about the lack of attention. She was frequently hopeless about changing her situation and would intermittently have suicidal thoughts of a pill overdose. She was guilt ridden and felt that she was "always screwing things up." During the course of treatment, described below, Ms. C received a series of medications, with moderate impact on her depressive symptoms.

Ms. C described a recurrent tendency to feel rejected by others, experiencing them either as not caring or as purposely malicious. She often felt enraged at what she perceived to be unjust treatment, especially by superiors or by those on whom she depended. These feelings alternated with a sense of herself as obese, bitter, and unlikable.

It became apparent during the initial interviews with Ms. C that her difficulties followed a particular pattern. She entered into relationships in a submissive and helping fashion, viewing herself as a person of little value who sought approval from a powerful, caring other. Over time, however, she would begin to feel unappreciated, misused, or overlooked. Ms. C would become frustrated and disappointed that the other person was not behaving in accord with her expectation of a loving caretaker. Feeling diminished and rejected, she would fear voicing her disappointment, out of anxiety that the other person would reject her further or confirm her suspicions that she was viewed as inadequate and undeserving.

In this context, Ms. C would act in a passive-aggressive manner. For instance, she would come late to meetings at her job or become withdrawn or sullen in her relationships. Often she was unaware of the hostility behind her behavior or of the potential impact of her sullen stance. In response to this hostile behavior, the individual with whom she was disappointed would often withdraw, and Ms. C would feel slighted. She would see herself as unjustly treated and wish for someone to rescue her and right the injustice that had occurred. Over time, however, she would become increasingly depressed and self-critical as the longed-for redressing of grievances did not occur. Her rage would become increasingly self-directed.

An example of this occurred in Ms. C's church, where she had been a very active member, often taking on many of the difficult volunteer duties. The patient idealized the church leaders as loving, caring men whose positive regard soothed her long-standing low self-esteem. However, she increasingly felt that the church leaders were not responsive to her problems with her husband, from whom she was later divorced. These problems included her husband's verbal abuse and criticisms. When the two of them met with the elders, she felt that they were siding with him and ignoring her concerns. She became angry but did not reveal her discontent to the church leaders. However, she appeared resentful and became derelict in her duties. The church leaders, increasingly frustrated with her behavior, eventually encouraged her to leave the parish. When Ms. C finally voiced her concerns, she did so with an abrasive bitterness that only alienated the clerics further.

Ms. C appealed her case to a higher church leader, convinced that he would redress her grievances. When this did not occur, she was extremely disappointed and plunged into a depressive state. She began to blame herself for these problems and felt her worthlessness and inadequacy were the source of her rejection by the church.

A similar series of events occurred at Ms. C's job, where she was shocked to receive a negative work review, reflecting her employer's dissatisfaction with a similar defiance and sullen withdrawal. Although she initially attributed the review's negativity to her boss's ignorance of her technical area, she became progressively more despondent, alternating between rage at him and criticism of herself as a failure.

Ms. C described growing up in an atmosphere of neglect in which she felt her parents were not interested in her and always busy with other things. Her mother was prickly and aggressive. In addition to intermittently screaming at Ms. C about her faults and imperfections, she would regularly engage in aggressive verbal attacks on others in the community. This led to constant disruptions of her mother's relationships and an isolated existence for the family. Her father, though more kind to her, was generally perceived as unavailable and either uninterested in or frightened about the idea of helping the patient deal with her mother. Ms. C was terrified of confronting her mother because she reported that when she had done so in the past, her mother would not speak to her for days, leaving her feeling helpless and needy.

Ms. C confided that it was important to her that she not behave like her mother, and she made every effort not to do so. This seemed to be one motivation for her shy, overly helpful behavior on initially meeting someone. She would view any attempts at self-assertion in a very critical fashion, associating such efforts with her mother's aggressive attacks on others. Ms. C also felt very guilty when she was angry, because she feared ripping others apart as she had seen her mother do. Ultimately, Ms. C would criticize herself for being like her mother when she became enraged at others, even though she expressed her hostility primarily in a passive manner.

Psychodynamic Models of Depression

Ms. C's depression can be explained by a variety of psychodynamic models, put forth by different psychoanalytic theorists (Table 2–1). Below, we apply each model to the case of Ms. C. We then use these theories to distill a set of psychodynamic factors central to the understanding and treatment of depression.

Early Psychoanalytic Models of Depression: Disappointment, Loss, and Anger

The first psychoanalytic writers to develop the concept that depression originates from narcissistic vulnerability, developmental traumas, and conflicted anger included Abraham (1911, 1924), Freud (1917), and Rado (1928).

Abraham (1911, 1924) provided an initial analytic framework for understanding depression when he described the syndrome as resulting from hostility toward others that becomes self-directed. Depressed patients with whom he worked demonstrated a propensity, based on temperament or early experiences, toward hatred and mistrust of others (Abraham 1911). Feeling unable to love the people with whom they are connected but frightened and guilty about their anger, such patients repress their hostility and project it externally. They begin to feel hated and then connect their sense of being disliked with various psychological or physical deficiencies: "People hate me because of these defects."

Abraham's description of his patients would be consistent with aspects of Ms. C's interpersonal dilemmas and subsequent depressions. Ms. C was troubled by persistent anger toward others, of which she was only minimally aware until it escalated. She would project this anger onto others and see them as hating her. Ms. C would then conclude that she must have a defect that would lead others to treat her this way. In addition, her perception of the world as a hateful place was disturbing and demoralizing.

Supplementing Abraham's initial observations on the dynamics of depression, Freud (1917) described an additional model for some cases. On the basis of his observations of similarities between bereavement and the depressed state, Freud hypothesized that the loss of an important person in the individual's life, either in reality or in fantasy, can trigger the onset of depression. As distinct from mourning, however, a depression is stimulated when the person who is lost has been the object of intensely ambivalent feelings

Table 2–1. Psychodynamic models of depression

Abraham

Predisposing factors	Traumatic early experiences; temperamental propensity toward aggressiveness, which becomes directed at others
Dynamic	Anger projected onto others, who are then experienced as hostile (patient concludes that he or she is inadequate, an object of scorn and hostility)

Freud

Predisposing factors	Perceived loss of someone for whom the patient experiences intensely ambivalent feelings
Dynamic	Identification with the lost other; anger toward the other comes to be directed toward the self

Rado

Predisposing factors	Narcissistic vulnerability: need for others to buttress self-esteem
Dynamic	"Good" aspects of the other internalized into superego, which attacks "bad" aspects internalized in the ego

Bibring

Predisposing factors	Frustration of a child's dependent needs
Dynamic	Discrepancy between the ego ideal (what one would like to be) and the view of the self

Jacobson

Predisposing factors	A lack of parental acceptance and emotional understanding; ambivalence toward others
Dynamic	Aggression toward disappointing parents that becomes self-directed to protect the loved other Internalized negative parental attitudes, leading to compensatory idealized expectation of self and others and recurrent disappointments

Stone

Predisposing factors	Disturbance of early childhood relationship with mother
Dynamic	Helplessness and frustration with this relationship, which generates reactive, coercive hostility and fuels a severe superego

Sandler and Joffe

Predisposing factors	Idealized relationship with a love object
Dynamic	Perceived or actual loss of this relationship, causing longing for the idealized state of being loved, and an experience of self-depletion leading to depression

Table 2–1.   Psychodynamic models of depression *(continued)*

Brenner

Predisposing factors   Heterogeneous factors, including those mentioned by other theorists

Dynamic   Expectation of castration or disempowerment for aggressive, competitive, or sexual wishes, triggering depression, with the resulting aggression directed toward self

Kohut

Predisposing factors   Traumatically unempathic experiences with early life caretakers, leading to narcissistic vulnerability

Dynamic   Unsuccessful efforts to idealize self and others to compensate for low self-esteem, leading to recurrent disappointments and depression

Bowlby

Predisposing factors   Disruptions of an adaptive attachment system from insecure and unstable relationships with parents

Dynamics   Internal models of the self as unlovable and inadequate, and others as unresponsive and punitive, triggered by loss or adversity

Fonagy and colleagues

Predisposing factors   Insecure attachment leading to disruptions in *mentalization,* the capacity to conceive and interpret behaviors and motives in self and others in terms of mental states

Dynamics   Insecure attachment and impaired or distorted mentalization, which increase the tendency to anticipate loss, failure, and rejection

on the part of the patient. The depressed individual identifies with, or takes on as part of himself or herself, one or another of the lost person's characteristics, to maintain a feeling of connection with that person and to mitigate against the sense of loss or bereavement. However, because the lost person was viewed with ambivalence, the anger originally directed toward that person now becomes directed toward the new attributes the patient has adopted. As a result, the patient begins to experience intense self-criticism and reproach, which eventually lead to depression.

In accord with Freud's theory of identification, when Ms. C identified herself with her mother's aggressive and hurtful behaviors toward others, she became extremely self-critical and felt worthless and unlovable. In Ms. C's case, however, the loss that connected most immediately with her current depression was that of her rapport with the previously idealized church leaders, not her mother. This can best be understood by Abraham's efforts to refine Freud's theory and make it consistent with his earlier model. Abraham (1924) came to view an episode of adult melancholia as stemming from a current disappointment in love, which is viewed, usually unconsciously, as a repetition of an early childhood traumatic experience.

Abraham (1924) posited that the depressed patient had had a severe injury to an early healthy sense of narcissism (self-esteem) by way of childhood disappointments in love, usually with the mother. Such an injury could stem, for example, from losing a view of the self as a parent's favorite or from disappointments in gaining an alliance with the mother against the father (or vice versa). Onset of the illness in adulthood is triggered by a new disappointment, unleashing strong hostile feelings toward those individuals, past and present, who have thwarted the patient's desire for love. For Ms. C, the church leaders she had relied on emotionally became the objects of considerable hostility once they disappointed her. Thus, she demonstrated a readiness to become enraged at those individuals, who, like her mother, had disappointed or neglected her. In fact, comments by Ms. C linked her anger at the leaders with her mother, as "people who preach one thing and behave completely differently."

Like Freud, Abraham posited that an identification with the rejecting person—past or present—leads to a pathological attack on the self. Once Ms. C experienced herself as having the same aggressive impulses as her mother had, she became immensely self-critical.

Rado (1928) amplified the theme of injured narcissism in depressed patients. He observed that his patients with depression had an intensely strong craving for others to buttress their self-esteem. He noted that accompanying this intense craving for narcissistic gratification was an intolerance of disappointment in the self or others. Thus, depressed patients reacted to trivial offenses and to failures in expectation not only with disappointment and anger but also with a significant fall in their self-esteem. They seemed wholly reliant on others to feel valued and valuable.

Ms. C resembles Rado's patients in this regard. Her depression connected not only to her sadness and anger about the clerics' presumed emotional unresponsiveness but also to her perception that her efforts within the church (and at work) were overlooked or underestimated. This contributed to the spiral of recriminations—against the church leaders and her boss and also against herself as being inadequate and without value. Thus, Ms. C attacked herself not only for being angry like her mother but also for seeming worthless to others and being unappreciated by them.

Adding to the theme of anger that becomes self-directed, Rado further described a split that takes place in the perception of self and others, in which the depressed patient sees the self or others as either all good or all bad. In the process of development of depression, the good qualities of the loved one are internalized in the patient's sense of whom he or she would like to be (or the ego ideal), whereas the bad qualities, as in Freud's formulation, become incorporated into the perception of the ego (or self). The self becomes the whipping boy of the superego, or the conscience function, which punishes the patient for failures to live up to the ego ideal. Thus, Ms. C internalized the self-righteousness of her mother in her superego and ego ideal, with the expectation that one should always behave with moral rectitude and kindness, and attacked herself for being unable to meet these standards.

Later Models for Depression: Problems With Self-Esteem Regulation and Aggression

Bibring (1953) followed Rado in his emphasis on the depressed patient's difficulties with feelings of narcissistic injury but differed with him and other analysts in what he saw as their overemphasis on matters of the superego and aggression. Instead, Bibring viewed depression as arising primarily from difficulties with self-esteem regulation. Low self-esteem, in this model, derives from a significant gap between the patient's self-view and what he or she would wish to be, or the ego ideal described in the previous subsection.

In Bibring's view, a primal experience of helplessness was most significant in contributing to the susceptibility to depression. Helplessness, which can develop from persistent frustration of a child's dependent needs, leads to a sense of failure and low self-esteem. Rather than anger toward others and subsequent guilt fueling the depression, helplessness triggers self-directed anger. A predisposition toward depression is seen by Bibring, then, as determined by a constitutional intolerance of frustration, by the severity and extent of situations of helplessness, and by later developmental factors that might confirm the patient's sense of self-disappointment and failure.

Seen from Bibring's point of view, Ms. C's low self-esteem stems from the discrepancy between her sense of herself as angry and hurtful like her mother and her ego ideal of being a very moral and caring person. She may have viewed this inadequacy as the cause of her father's disinclination to help her and of her mother's perceived neglect. A sense of helplessness about capturing their recognition stimulated significant anger toward herself not only as a deflection of her rage and disappointment toward her parents but also out of a sense of frustration and contempt toward herself for her inability to capture their love.

Jacobson (1954, 1971, 1975) offered an alternative approach to considering self-esteem regulation in the depressed patient. She posited a lack of parental acceptance and emotional understanding that diminishes the child's self-esteem, leading to ambivalence, aggressive feelings toward the parents, and guilt. This aggression is turned against the self as a defensive strategy to protect the loved person and to prevent the self from enacting hostile impulses toward the external world. Jacobson believed that to further counteract the negative impact of parental attitudes, the depressed patient develops an excessively perfectionistic reactive ego ideal and an excessively strict superego. The patient blames himself or herself for any attitudes or behaviors that resemble those despised and feared in the parents. Loved ones are idealized as part of the strategy of protecting them from aggression and supporting the patient's fragile self-esteem. This idealization leads the depressed individual to expect others to do more than they realistically can, leading to recurrent disappointments. Thus, the dependency on an overvalued other and the presence of excessively high self-expectations lead to an unstable and diminished sense of self-esteem and to narcissistic vulnerability.

Applying Jacobson's formulation to the case of Ms. C further clarifies the types of interpersonal relationships that contribute to her susceptibility toward depressive episodes. Namely, she idealizes others to support her fragile self-esteem and mute her anger. This idealization, however, inevitably leads to disappointment in those on whom she depends. Her anger in response to this disappointment triggers guilt, as it reminds her of her volatile mother, lowering her self-esteem. She fails to live up to her overly perfectionistic self-expectations, and her shame about this adds to her depressive affect.

Stone (1986) highlighted particularly the reactive aggression that develops in a deeply frustrating early relationship between the person who later develops depression and his or her parent. The aggression becomes expressed in repeated, failed attempts to coerce the parent to respond to his or her needs. A severe superego develops, fueled by the helpless anger.

Following Stone's model, a therapist might explore extensively with Ms. C nuances in her historical relationship with her mother, compassionately highlighting her efforts to coerce this seemingly unresponsive parent, and then others, into recognizing and addressing her needs. This approach might help the patient recognize her hostility and its impact on others and find alternate avenues for expressing her disappointments.

Sandler and Joffe (1965) researched the extensive case files of the Hampstead Clinic to look for dynamic trends in their child patients showing evidence of depressive syndromes. These authors found that the depressive reaction seemed to occur most often when children felt that they had lost something essential to their self-esteem and felt helpless to undo the loss. Typically, this was the loss of an important loved one in reality or fantasy, and especially of a state of well-being implicit in the relationship with that person. This state of well-being tends to become idealized: The more it is elevated and longed for, the greater will be the depressive reaction in the face of its unattainability. Working with their model, one might emphasize with Ms. C the loss of her sense of well-being that existed when she felt supported by the clerics and pleased with her sense of accomplishment at work, and focus on her depression as representing a yearning to return to that state.

Rather than focusing on loss as a trigger for depression, Brenner (1975, 1979) saw many of his patients as imagining themselves to be decisively disempowered, or symbolically castrated, by others as a punishment for competitive, sexual, and aggressive wishes. Thus, actual or fantasized successes could be a trigger of depression via the need for punishment, and depression could be a means of diminishing a more effective, competitive stance. Aggression is mobilized against the person blamed for creating this disempowerment but becomes self-directed as the patient begins to adopt an ingratiating or propitiatory stance toward the blamed but feared party.

Using Brenner's perspective, a therapist would attempt to discern for which childhood wishes—sexual, competitive, aggressive—Ms. C may have felt that she had been punished, causing her to experience herself as a helpless, powerless individual overlooked and unloved by all. In fact, this patient's childhood concerns about competitive feelings toward her mother for her father's attention and her apparent fear of punishment by her mother were seen by her therapist as significant in the evolution of her guilty inhibitions.

Kohut (1971) wrote extensively about patients' problems with narcissistic injury and was particularly interested in issues of technique in engaging and treating such patients. According to Kohut, depressive affects in narcissistically vulnerable individuals are related to chronic feelings of emptiness, in response to traumatically unempathic parenting. When children's affective experiences are not sensitively mirrored by their primary caretakers, they are left feeling alone with their experience and emotionally empty, and they struggle to fill themselves by finding others to idealize and identify with. Rather than a realistic sense of themselves and their capabilities, they develop a compensatory grandiose sense of self that persists into adulthood. However, recurrent disappointments will trigger the underlying low self-esteem. Technical attention to mirroring these patients' feelings and to issues of idealization and devaluation in the transference relationship with the therapist are emphasized (Kohut 1971). Ms. C's treatment, described in Chapter 3 ("Overview of Psychodynamic Psychotherapy for Depression") in this volume, was enhanced by her therapist's attention to this patient's hunger for recognition and empathy. A need to idealize the therapist was not confronted initially. However, the therapist suggested that it was important to be alert to disappointments and that she should feel safe addressing those with him.

Attachment Theory

Attachment theory, as developed by Bowlby (1969, 1980), draws heavily on an ethological and adaptational perspective and has had a significant influence on psychoanalytic models of psychopathology. Bowlby viewed attachment as a behavioral system essential for survival, and disruptions of attachment, such as loss of a parent, as crucial in the etiology of anxious and depressive disorders. Loss triggers a series of responses: angry protest, anxiety, mourning, and ultimately, detachment. Disrupted attachments due to insecure and unstable relationships with parents, or to their rejecting and critical behavior, lead to the development of internal models of the self as unlovable and inadequate and of others as unresponsive and punitive. The individual becomes vulnerable to depression in the setting of later experiences of loss or adversity, seeing such losses as signs of failure and expecting little support from others.

Although Ms. C did not lose a parent early in life, her experience of disrupted attachment from critical and emotionally unresponsive parents clearly contributed to her view of herself as inadequate and helpless to change complex and adverse situations. The loss of the church intensified feelings of failure, helpless rage, and hopelessness about her ability to have successful attachments to others. For example, Ms. C thought it was useless to look for a new church because it would invariably lead to another failure.

Others psychoanalysts have subsequently explored the impact of insecure and disrupted attachment on cognition and emotion. Fonagy and colleagues

(Fonagy and Target 1997) have focused on the adverse impact of insecure attachment on the development of *mentalization,* the ability to conceive of behavior and motives in the self and others in terms of mental states. A disruption or distortion in this capacity, in the context of insecure attachment, can lead to problems with affect regulation and expectations of loss, failure, and rejection. These expectations can adversely affect relationships. Preliminary studies suggest that depressed patients suffer from a deficit in mentalization (Fischer-Kern et al. 2008, 2013). The capacity to better recognize the motives and emotional states of self and others can aid patients in understanding negative reactions of others and experiencing them less personally. Ms. C had difficulty mentalizing about the motives of others, frequently presuming that their main intention was to deliberately judge or attack her. However, as she developed mentalizing capacities, she was more able to recognize that other factors may be influencing their attitudes and behavior. For instance, she was able to identify that her boss was under pressure to meet deadlines imposed by his supervisors and that this pressure contributed to his increased criticism of her. This helped her to feel less vulnerable and to better understand his criticisms and take them less personally.

Defense Mechanisms in Depression

Psychoanalytic theorists have considered the possibility that certain defenses (i.e., internal or behavioral means of averting painful feelings or threatening unconscious fantasies) either may be specifically mobilized by depressive affects or may predispose individuals to the development of depressive syndromes (Brenner 1975; Jacobson 1971).

Bloch et al. (1993) described three possibilities in this regard: 1) defenses may become structured in response to a chronic mood disturbance; 2) maladaptive defenses may actually lead to depression; and 3) the mood disorder and defenses may each be related to a third factor, such as underlying low self-esteem. For most theoreticians, the defenses in depressed patients are initially triggered to contend with intolerably angry fantasies or with painfully low self-esteem but actually only result in an exacerbation of depression. Thus, anger projected outward, according to Abraham (1911), ends up being directed toward the self, whereas efforts to idealize the self or others to cope with low self-esteem eventually lead only to further disappointment and devaluation (Jacobson 1971). Other defenses mentioned specifically by psychoanalytic authors as mobilized to cope with intolerable anger and sadness include denial, passive aggression, reaction formation, and identification with the aggressor.

In a more systematic study by Bloch et al. (1993), the defense mechanisms employed by patients with dysthymic disorder were compared with those of patients with panic disorder, by using the Defense Mechanism Rating Scale (DMRS) (Perry 1990). The scale, which contains criteria for operationalized assessment for the presence or absence of each defense, is scored by use of a psychodynamic interview. Two defenses, denial and repression, were found to be used frequently by both patients with panic disorder and patients with dysthymia. Compared with panic disorder patients, those with dysthymia were found to employ higher levels of devaluation, passive aggression, projection, hypochondriasis, acting out, and projective identification. In the formulation by Bloch et al. (1993) from the data, depression could occur through directing anger toward the self, expressing anger passively (passive aggression), distorting perceptions of self and others (devaluation, projection), inviting retaliation from others (acting out, passive aggression), or asking for and then rejecting help (related to the DMRS formulation for hypochondriasis). Although there has been variability in results (Porcerelli et al. 2009), subsequent studies have generally substantiated the increased presence of these defenses in depressive disorders (Høglend and Perry 1998).

In individual patients, the clinician should be alert to the characteristic defenses that they employ, particularly to those noted above (see Chapter 10, "Defense Mechanisms in Depressed Patients," in this volume). Feedback to patients about the nature and impact of these defenses may allow them to more effectively cope with their feelings and alter their characteristic perceptions of and responses toward others. In the case of Ms. C, her initial presentation included the defenses of passive aggression, repressed anger, the projection of her anger onto others, and identification with the aggressor, via her guilty identifications with her mother's rage.

Parental Perceptions of Depressed Patients

To test the suggestions of many theorists that problematic parental behavior may contribute to the development of depression, some researchers have explored patients' perceptions of parents by use of systematic assessment instruments. Using the parental bonding instrument, Parker (1983) found that depressed patients viewed their parents as having less emotional warmth and as being more protective than did a control group without depressive disorders. In a study by Perris et al. (1986), patients with depressive disorders were compared with healthy control subjects by using the EMBU, a Swedish instrument for assessing parental perceptions. The authors found that depressed patients experienced less emotional warmth from their parents, but they did not find prominent experiences of overprotection. The authors concluded that "rearing practices which deprived the child of love might be an important risk factor predisposing to depression" (p. 174). MacKinnon et al. (1993) also found that the experience of neglectful care, rather than overprotection, was the more significant factor. Although depressed mood could cause a retrospective distortion of memories of parents, studies suggest that improvement in depression does not affect these perceptions (Gerlsma et al. 1993; Gotlib et al. 1988; Parker 1981; Plantes et al. 1988; Nitta et al. 2008).

These studies are consistent with the notions suggested by Abraham, Bowlby, and others that early traumatic injuries experienced with parents predispose to the development of depression. Alternatively, patients may perceive their parents as being uncaring or rejecting because of their own predisposition to feeling rejected. In either case, it is crucial that such internal parental representations be explored to gain an understanding of the patient's depression.

Central Dynamics of Depression: A Summary

Several core dynamics of depression have been identified by these theoreticians (Table 2–2).

Despite their variations in focus, almost all psychoanalysts describing their patients with depression have emphasized narcissistic vulnerability as triggering susceptibility to this syndrome. The basis of this vulnerability varies, however, from disappointments in early relationships to fragile self-esteem based on factors such as childhood experiences of helplessness or reactive fantasies of disempowerment or castration. A sense of narcissistic injury predisposes patients toward the experience of shame and anger, which may become important aspects or triggers of later depressive episodes.

Theorists also focus on conflicted anger as playing a key role in the dynamics of depression, although the origin of the anger and the form it takes

---

Table 2–2.　Central dynamics of depression

Narcissistic vulnerability

Cause	Early experience or perceptions of loss, rejection, inadequacy, possible biochemical vulnerability
Content	Sensitivity to perceived or actual losses, rejections
Consequences	Recurrent lowering of self-esteem, triggering depressive affects; rage in response to experience of injury

Conflicted anger

Cause	Response to narcissistic injury; anger at perceived or actual lack of responsiveness of others to the individual's needs and wishes; anger may also arise from a blaming of others for one's sense of vulnerability, or being deeply envious of those who seem less vulnerable
Content	Anger at others for injurious, unresponsive behavior, attitudes; blaming others for one's vulnerability; envy of others who are viewed as less vulnerable; anger at others experienced as damaging, threatening, unacceptable, requiring suppression or redirection
Consequences	Disruptions in interpersonal relationships; anger turned toward the self, triggering depressive affects, lowering of self-esteem

Severe superego, experience of guilt and shame

Cause	Anger turned toward the self via harsh self-judgments; internalization of parental attitudes perceived as harsh and punitive
Content	Anger, greed, envy, sexuality, and accompanying wishes seen as wrong or bad
Consequences	Negative self-perceptions and self-criticisms trigger lowering of self-esteem, depressive affects

Idealized and devalued expectations of self, others

Cause	Efforts to mitigate low self-esteem
Content	High self-expectations (ego ideal), others idealized in meeting individual's needs, others devalued to bolster self-esteem
Consequences	Significant disappointment, anger at self and others, with lowering of self-esteem

Table 2–2.   Central dynamics of depression *(continued)*

Characteristic means of defending against painful affects (defenses)

Cause	Intolerable feelings of low self-esteem, anger
Content	Denial, projection (seeing anger as coming from others), passive aggression (expressing anger indirectly), reaction formation (denial of anger accompanied by compensatory overly positive feelings)
Consequences	Anger not effectively dealt with; increased depression via anger directed toward the self or via world seen as hostile, menacing, uncaring, or defeating

may vary. In general the anger is seen as triggered by narcissistic injury, loss, immense frustration, or a sense of helplessness. In many of the models explored earlier in this chapter, aggression triggers conscious or unconscious guilt, which contributes to the self-punishing aspects of the patient's mood, the tendency to self-denigration, and self-defeating behaviors that reinforce the depressive cycle.

In almost every theorist's description, aggression ultimately is directed toward the self, although the basis of this dynamic varies. The possibilities include hatred projected outward and then experienced as directed toward the self, and aggressive feelings and fantasies directed toward aspects of the self identified with an ambivalently experienced other. A severe superego attacks the self for various aggressive, competitive, and sexual feelings, lowering self-esteem.

Several authors have referred to attempts to modulate self-esteem and aggression via idealization and devaluation, leading to increased susceptibility to depression when idealized others prove to be disappointing. Multiple authors also have emphasized an overly perfectionistic ego ideal and superego in their depressed patients. Patients fail to live up to their narcissistic aspirations and moral expectations, leading to a loss of self-esteem.

Finally, characteristic defenses, such as denial, projection, passive aggression, and reaction formation, are described as a means of warding off painful depressive affects but often result in a further lowering of self-esteem.

A Core Dynamic Formulation for Depression

The literature, then, suggests two broad models of depression: those involving aggression toward others that is ultimately directed toward the self,

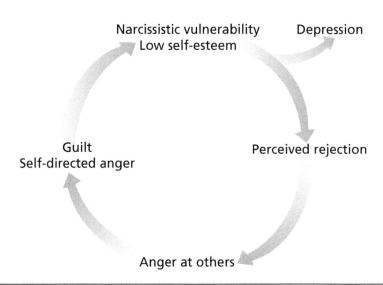

Figure 2–1. Vicious cycle 1 in depression: narcissistic vulnerability and anger.

and those focusing on difficulties with self-esteem in patients whose expectations of themselves and others far exceed the capacity to live up to them. Finally, some theorists refer to links between the two models.

These factors can be integrated into two core dynamic formulations for depression, which can trigger vicious cycles (Busch et al. 2004; Rudden et al. 2003). In each formulation, narcissistic vulnerability and low self-esteem are seen as fundamental to the susceptibility to depression. In depression cycle 1 (Figure 2–1), this vulnerability results in sensitivity to disappointment and rejection and thus to easily triggered rage, which leads to feelings of guilt and worthlessness. The self-directed rage compounds the injury to an individual's self-esteem, which then escalates the narcissistic vulnerability, and so on, in a vicious cycle. Defenses, including denial, projection, passive aggression, identification with the aggressor, and reaction formation, are triggered in an attempt to diminish these painful feelings but result in an intensification of depression. Precipitants for depression in this integrative model can include either perceived or actual loss or rejection, the failure to live up to a perfectionistic ego ideal, and superego punishment for sexual and aggressive fantasies.

Another core dynamic in depression (depression cycle 2) is the individual's attempt to deal with low self-esteem by idealization and devaluation (Figure 2–2). A depressive state will lead to compensatory idealization of self

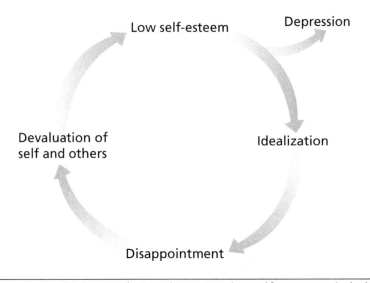

Figure 2–2. Vicious cycle 2 in depression: low self-esteem and idealization/devaluation.

or others, increasing the likelihood and intensity of eventual disappointment, triggering depression. An ego ideal with highly unrealistic standards develops, increasing the level of disappointment with and devaluation of the self when the standards cannot be met. The disappointment leads to feelings of self-directed anger. Alternately, individuals may devalue others to maintain self-esteem, but the aggression in this stance triggers superego punishment. In addition, aggressive behavior may lead to the patient's alienating others, adding to feelings of abandonment and rejection. The two sets of dynamics also interact with each other, because conflicts over self-esteem and anger can heighten the tendency to idealization and devaluation, and disappointments following idealization can lead to anger, guilt, and self-criticism. Although these cycles represent core dynamics of depression, clinicians should not restrict themselves to these factors and should remain alert to other areas of vulnerability, intrapsychic conflict, and defense.

As described earlier in this chapter, the case of Ms. C demonstrates these dynamics. Treatment approaches that were helpful in overcoming her major depression and in substantially reversing her dysthymia are discussed in Chapter 3 in this volume, which provides an overview of the psychodynamic treatment of depression.

References

Abraham K: Notes on the psycho-analytical investigation and treatment of manic-depressive insanity and allied conditions (1911), in Selected Papers on Psychoanalysis. London, Hogarth Press, 1927, pp 137–156

Abraham K: A short study of the development of the libido, viewed in the light of mental disorders (1924), in Selected Papers on Psychoanalysis. London, Hogarth Press, 1927, pp 418–501

Bibring E: The mechanics of depression, in Affective Disorders: Psychoanalytic Contributions to Their Study. Edited by Greenacre P. New York, International Universities Press, 1953, pp 13–48

Bloch AL, Shear MK, Markowitz JC, et al: An empirical study of defense mechanisms in dysthymia. Am J Psychiatry 150(8):1194–1198, 1993 8328563

Bowlby J: Attachment and Loss, Vol 1: Attachment. New York, Basic Books, 1969

Bowlby J: Attachment and Loss, Vol 3: Loss. New York, Basic Books, 1980

Brenner C: Affects and psychic conflict. Psychoanal Q 44(1):5–28, 1975 1114198

Brenner C: Depressive affect, anxiety, and psychic conflict in the phallic-oedipal phase. Psychoanal Q 48(2):177–197, 1979 441209

Busch FN, Rudden MG, Shapiro T: Psychodynamic Treatment of Depression. Washington, DC, American Psychiatric Press, 2004

Fischer-Kern M, Tmej A, Kapusta ND, et al: The capacity for mentalization in depressive patients: a pilot study. Z Psychosom Med Psychother 54:368–380, 2008 19049686

Fischer-Kern M, Fonagy P, Kapusta ND, et al: Mentalizing in female inpatients with major depressive disorder. J Nerv Ment Dis 201:202–207, 2013 23407204

Fonagy P, Target M: Attachment and reflective function: their role in self-organization. Dev Psychopathol 9(4):679–700, 1997 9449001

Freud S: Mourning and melancholia (1917), in The Standard Edition of the Complete Psychological Works of Sigmund Freud, Vol 14. Translated and edited by Strachey J. London, Hogarth Press, 1957, pp 239–258

Gerlsma C, Das J, Emmelkamp PM: Depressed patients' parental representations: stability across changes in depressed mood and specificity across diagnoses. J Affect Disord 27(3):173–181, 1993 8478505

Gotlib IH, Mount JH, Cordy NI, Whiffen VE: Depression and perceptions of early parenting: a longitudinal investigation. Br J Psychiatry 152:24–27, 1988 3167341

Høglend P, Perry JC: Defensive functioning predicts improvement in major depressive episodes. J Nerv Ment Dis 186(4):238–243, 1998 9569892

Jacobson E: Transference problems in the psychoanalytic treatment of severely depressed patients. J Am Psychoanal Assoc 2:695–705, 1954

Jacobson E: Depression: Comparative Studies of Normal, Neurotic, and Psychotic Conditions. New York, International Universities Press, 1971

Jacobson E: The psychoanalytic treatment of depressive patients, in Depression and Human Existence. Edited by Anthony B. Boston, MA, Little, Brown, 1975, pp 431–443

Kohut H: The Analysis of the Self. New York, International Universities Press, 1971

MacKinnon A, Henderson AS, Andrews G: Parental 'affectionless control' as an antecedent to adult depression: a risk factor refined. Psychol Med 23(1):135–141, 1993 8475201

Nitta M, Narita T, Umeda K, et al: Influence of negative cognition on the parental bonding instrument (PBI) in patients with major depression. J Nerv Ment Dis 196(3):244–246, 2008 18340261

Parker G: Parental reports of depressives. An investigation of several explanations. J Affect Disord 3(2):131–140, 1981 6454707

Parker G: Parental 'affectionless control' as an antecedent to adult depression. A risk factor delineated. Arch Gen Psychiatry 40(9):956–960, 1983 6615158

Perris C, Arrindell WA, Perris H, et al: Perceived depriving parental rearing and depression. Br J Psychiatry 148:170–175, 1986 3697584

Perry JC: The Defense Mechanism Rating Scales, 5th Edition. Cambridge, MA, Author, 1990

Plantes MM, Prusoff BA, Brennan J, Parker G: Parental representations of depressed outpatients from a U.S.A. sample. J Affect Disord 15(2):149–155, 1988 2975685

Porcerelli JH, Olson TR, Presniak MD, et al: Defense mechanisms and major depressive disorder in African American women. J Nerv Ment Dis 197(10):736–741, 2009 19829201

Rado S: The problem of melancholia. Int J Psychoanal 9:420–438, 1928

Rudden M, Busch FN, Milrod B, et al: Panic disorder and depression: a psychodynamic exploration of comorbidity. Int J Psychoanal 84(Pt 4):997–1015, 2003 13678503

Sandler J, Joffe WG: Notes on childhood depression. Int J Psychoanal 46:88–96, 1965 14289320

Stone L: Psychoanalytic observations on the pathology of depressive illness: selected spheres of ambiguity or disagreement. J Am Psychoanal Assoc 34(2):329–362, 1986 3722700

Overview of Psychodynamic Psychotherapy for Depression

IN psychodynamic psychotherapy for depression, the therapist maintains a continued focus on understanding depressive symptoms, gradually linking these to the core depressive dynamics delineated in Chapter 2 ("Development of a Psychodynamic Model of Depression") of this volume. As the treatment progresses, the patient achieves greater insight into the ways in which these dynamics have become the scaffolding for self-perceptions and aspects of relationships with others. During the middle and termination phases of the treatment, there is opportunity to explore the manifestations of these conflicts in multiple and varied circumstances, including in the relationship with the therapist. Gradually, the patient begins to recognize the contexts that tend to elicit depression, to understand what is happening internally during these times, and to feel more in control of the depressed feelings.

The treatment of Ms. C, whose case illustrated the various core dynamics of depressive disorders in Chapter 2, is briefly described here to provide an overview of actual psychodynamic therapy for depression.

Elements of the initial evaluation of depression are discussed in Chapter 1 ("Introduction") of this volume. In this chapter, we provide an overview of the phases of treatment, and each is addressed in greater detail in Part II

("Techniques in Psychodynamic Treatment of Depression") of this volume. Tables 3–1, 3–2, and 3–3 illustrate these three treatment phases.

Phase 1: Forming a Therapeutic Alliance and a Frame for Treatment

As seen in Table 3–1, phase 1 of this treatment is characterized by an initial examination of the depressive symptoms and the context in which they have occurred. The therapist establishes a safe base of cooperation in which he or she helps patients to understand that their depressive symptoms have meaning, and are affected by their experience of current and past relationships and events, and their struggles about feelings and fantasies. The therapist works collaboratively with the patient to uncover a developmental under- standing of the depressed feelings and the fantasies that accompany them within the patient's history, to identify particular areas of conflict that seem to trigger the depressed feelings currently, and to begin understanding the meanings of each of the patient's particular depressive ideas. Within this collaboration, the therapist and patient form an alliance, ideally with the therapist perceived as both a sympathetic and nonjudgmental collaborator in understanding, and as an authoritative voice with knowledge about and experience in treating the patient's illness. In this phase, as the therapist ex- plores the patient's symptoms, he or she begins to develop a dynamic formu- lation that specifically integrates the patient's experiences and perceptions with the core dynamics described in our model. The patient's recognition of the value of exploring the meanings, context, and dynamics of symptoms aids in building the therapeutic alliance. The patient gradually feels relief from depression in the context of a hopeful, affectively charged relationship with the therapist, and as the symptoms begin to feel understandable and thus potentially manageable.

In the treatment of Ms. C, the initial phase focused on identifying her symptoms, such as a sense of being a bad person and feeling helpless to pre- vent rejection or attack by others, and the contexts in which they intensified (i.e., being expelled from her church). This helped Ms. C to gain a sense that her symptoms had meaning and were related to her internal states and interpersonal experiences. The therapist helped her to see how she rapidly came to interpret problems arising in the course of her work and church relationships as evidence that she was globally impaired, flawed and "bad," rather than as evidence of more discrete and manageable difficulties. These

Table 3–1.   Phase 1: beginning of treatment

The therapist examines the depressive symptoms and their context with the patient to uncover developmental determinants, identify areas of intrapsychic conflict, and begin understanding the meanings of the symptoms.

Areas of focus

1. Establishing the treatment frame and engaging the patient in a therapeutic alliance
2. Exploring the symptoms, stressors, perceptions, and feelings accompanying the onset of depression. Identifying ways in which these factors are related to depression.
3. Linking item 2 above to the core dynamics for depression, in the present and during the patient's development:
   a. Narcissistic vulnerability based on experiences/perceptions of loss, illness, rejection, separation, or difference
   b. Reactive, conflicted anger (including feelings of envy, blame, jealousy, vengeance), often ultimately directed toward the self
   c. Guilt resulting from anger; shame, resulting from a sense of inadequacy or damage related to the experiences or perceptions mentioned in item 3a
   d. Compensatory idealization of self or others, followed by disappointment and devaluation
   e. Defenses employed in coping with painful affects

Expected responses

1. Reduction in depressive symptoms
2. Tentative formulation offered to the patient of central themes and dynamisms
3. Establishment of a good working relationship

perceptions were linked to her feelings about herself from her childhood relationships with her mother, in which she had often felt helpless and disappointing, and her father, in which she had never felt "special" enough to draw him into a meaningful relationship. Ms. C began to realize how much she anticipated and expected others' criticism by examining her reaction to even supportive comments made by her therapist as if they were judgmental. Through this exploration, Ms. C realized that she spent so much time defending herself against others' imagined criticisms that it was difficult for her to relax and enjoy her relationships with others and that instead, she distanced herself from people. This invariably led to the anticipated "rejection" when others, not understanding her behavior, withdrew from her.

During the early phase of her treatment, Ms. C also became aware of how angry she had been toward her mother, whom she had experienced as deeply frustrating, unresponsive, and critical. She developed a preliminary recognition that her anger invariably led to vicious self-attacks, in part because anger reminded Ms. C of her mother, whom she felt was unacceptably aggressive and judgmental, and in part because her anger triggered intense feelings of guilt and shame (see depression cycle 1 [Figure 2–1] in Chapter 2, "Development of a Psychodynamic Model of Depression"). In this context, Ms. C began to recognize how her symptoms could be triggered by her own intrapsychic conflicts about her feelings and fantasies.

Phase 2: Treatment of Vulnerability to Depression

In the middle phase of treatment, the therapist focuses on understanding the patient's particular vulnerability to depressive symptoms (Table 3–2). The individual version of core depressive dynamics is explored and understood from as many vantage points as possible, as the patient has experienced these dynamics internally and in fantasy, in relation to significant others in the present and past, and in their emergence in the transference relationship with the therapist. The deeper understanding that results from this continued collaboration allows the patient to more easily identify the depressive constellations when they emerge and to experience a greater sense of control in recognizing and managing them.

In the middle phase of her treatment, Ms. C accomplished a good deal of work in recognizing how an exquisite sense of helplessness in the face of others' expectations and a sense of herself as always potentially disappointing contributed to her depression and to her continual defensiveness with others. She recognized the often passive expressions of her anger and realized how deeply she feared directly expressing angry feelings because of her terror of rejection, which was based on her mother's tendency to respond to any complaint of hers with a prolonged, silent withdrawal. She gradually came to understand how disruptive the indirect expression of her rage was in her relationships with her boss and in her church. Ms. C also became more able to distinguish her own anger from that of her mother and to realize that her own behaviors, although problematic, did not deserve the same level of self-censure as did her mother's very destructive and vicious attacks toward others. She gradually became more able to directly express angry feel-

Table 3–2.   Phase 2: middle of treatment

To reduce the vulnerability to depression, the dynamisms described in the text are understood from many vantage points, as the patient has experienced them internally and in fantasy, in relation to significant others in the present and past, and in their emergence with the therapist. Greater understanding permits easier identification of depressive constellations when they emerge and a greater sense of control in managing them.

Areas of focus
1.   Addressing conflicted feelings and fantasies related to the central dynamics, as they emerge with significant others in the present and past
2.   Addressing related feelings and fantasies in the transference
3.   Greater understanding of and control over these conflicts by exploring their presence in a variety of forms and contexts

Expected responses
1.   Reduced vulnerability of self-esteem to loss, disappointments, criticism
2.   Increased tolerance of anger accompanied by greater recognition of this affect, and of the tendency to turn it against the self
3.   Reduction in guilt and self-punishing behaviors
4.   Improved interpersonal relationships, less contaminated by shame and by idealization/devaluation

ings in a moderated fashion, including toward the therapist, and see that they might be helpful in improving a relationship rather than causing an attack or disruption.

Ms. C was gradually able to see that her passively expressed anger toward her boss also stemmed from a need to devalue him in order to bolster a sense of her own worth, a realization that was quite painful for her. She was able to fully grasp it after work in the transference on her tendency to devalue her therapist when she felt particularly vulnerable herself. This occurred, for example, at times of separation, such as vacations, when she would view the therapist as "not caring," and experience his departure as a rejection.

Finally, work in the middle phase of this patient's treatment focused a good deal on her distortions of others as critical and frustrating, alternating with occasionally seeing some people, such as the elders of her church, in an excessively idealized way. This idealization would often give way to excruciating disappointment followed by depression when the idealized others failed to meet her extremely high standards and she no longer felt protected or specially cared for by them (see depression cycle 2 [Figure 2–2] in Chapter 2).

Ms. C was able to see these cycles of idealization and devaluation in her reactions to her therapist, and she gradually learned to assess her relationships more realistically. As this work was accomplished in her treatment, Ms. C was able to recognize when her mood began to become somewhat low and to talk herself through it by understanding and then managing her feelings better.

Phase 3: Termination

During the termination phase, the patient often experiences a sense of loss related to the ending of the deepened relationship with the therapist (Table 3–3). The patient may also become angry that the relationship is ending or about perceived limitations of work in therapy. This loss and anger may stimulate a brief recurrence of depressive symptoms, which can be understood in an affectively charged and meaningful manner with the therapist. Experiencing, observing, and understanding the unique ways in which the patient perceives the loss and the anger and observing the ways in which these perceptions may trigger depressive feelings are very useful. At this point in treatment, the patient can observe and articulate feelings to a much greater degree and becomes aware of possessing the tools to relieve sadness and distress.

In the termination phase, despite an agreed-on plan to end treatment, Ms. C experienced her therapist as abandoning her, leaving her to manage difficult feelings on her own. She became aware of how much the end of therapy reminded her of sad and resentful feelings she had about her father's withdrawal from her life. Anger at her therapist for his perceived abandonment led to an increased understanding of how her anger intensified the threat that she would be rejected. The recognition of these feelings offered Ms. C a greater opportunity to work on dynamics that she had realized were crucial to her depressive experience.

Table 3–3.   Phase 3: termination of treatment

Termination provides a crucial opportunity for further work with the dynamics of depression, especially as they emerge in the transference.

Areas of focus

1. Understanding feelings about the loss of the therapist and the ending of treatment
2. Coping with the sense of narcissistic injury in fantasies of a continued relationship with the therapist
3. Anger with the therapist over termination and the limitations of treatment

Expected responses

1. Possible briefly intensified depressive symptoms as termination approaches and the patient contends with a powerful resurgence of feelings about loss and separation
2. Increased capacity to cope with loss and narcissistic injury
3. More effective use of anger with less self-direction
4. Reduced guilt and need for self-punishment

II PART

Techniques in Psychodynamic Treatment of Depression

CHAPTER 4

Getting Started With Psychodynamic Treatment of Depression

IN the initial treatment phase (Table 4–1), a therapeutic alliance is formed and the particular frame for a psychodynamic treatment is established. The patient is introduced to the idea that symptoms have meaning and are triggered by events in the present that evoke unpleasant affective experiences and the fantasies linked with them in the past. In this regard, it can be mentioned, if it seems helpful to the patient, that our emphasis on the past is intended not to blame parents or others but rather to learn how the patient might have understood family relationships from a childhood vantage. The continuing effects of these powerful perceptions about self and others contributing to depression, and usually maintained out of the patient's awareness, can be modified by bringing them into conscious adult perspective. In addition, patients gain a sense that they are in conflict about certain feelings and fantasies, such as vengeful wishes toward an important attachment figure. These conflicts can trigger guilt and self-criticism that intensify depressive symptoms.

In this phase, the central dynamic factors contributing to depression are identified and explored as they apply to each patient:

1. Areas of narcissistic vulnerability and shame stemming from experiences of loss, separation, rejection, or illness

2. Difficulties in managing conflicts about the reactive anger connected with these experiences, including identifying the tendency to direct it toward oneself
3. Identification of guilty reactions to the range of angry affects, including greed, envy, vengefulness, and competitiveness, and to sexual desires
4. Tendency to idealize and devalue self and others
5. Characteristic ways the patient defends against the painful affects stimulated by loss and rejection

Establishing the Therapeutic Frame

As the recommendation for dynamic psychotherapy is made, it is important to introduce its basic format and to connect each aspect explicitly with how it will help the patient's depressive symptoms. The therapist can review and describe the patient's depressive symptoms and provide education about the potential neurobiological and psychological contributions to depression. The psychological attitudes about self and others and the ways in which the patient understands and manages painful affects are identified as the focus for exploration.

For a genuine exploratory process to develop, dynamic psychotherapy is best accomplished with a minimum of twice-weekly sessions (Dewald 1996). Weekly visits may be adequate, however, if the patient 1) is particularly psychologically minded, or quickly develops this capacity; 2) is able to maintain an affective connection and focus on the work; and 3) does not need the concrete contact with the therapist for support. It is important to clarify policies about billing and missed sessions from the outset of treatment. It can be noted that repetitive behaviors such as late payment, frequent lateness to sessions, or spotty attendance may provide clues to other ways in which the patient expresses and manages painful, depressive feelings and will be explored as such.

Introducing the Concepts of Free Association and Transference

Patients are encouraged to say whatever comes to mind, even if it seems hurtful or trivial, because following one's train of thoughts is very important in this type of treatment. This is the concept of free association, which attempts to explore the mind's multiple associative links to a symptom, in the

---

Table 4–1.   Initial treatment phase

I. Establishing the therapeutic frame

    A. Treatment frequency, billing policies

    B. Introducing the exploratory process

        1. Free association and the transference

        2. Meaning of symptoms

II. Establishing the therapeutic alliance

    A. Therapist as nonjudgmental, sympathetic partner in exploration

    B. Therapist as knowledgeable authority (early identification of meaning and context of symptoms can aid in developing the alliance)

III. Identifying barriers to engagement in treatment

    A. Excessive shame and fear of exposure

    B. Excessive guilt

    C. Overvalued explanations for depression

IV. Clarifying the central depressive psychodynamics; suggesting a preliminary formulation of the dynamics

    A. Narcissistic vulnerability and shame

    B. Managing conflicted anger and anger directed toward the self

    C. Excessive guilt

    D. Idealization and devaluation

    E. Defenses employed in coping with painful affects

---

expectation that through this process, over time, the often divergent contributions to that symptom will be better understood (Kris 1962; Meissner 2000). Also, this process aids in revealing fantasies and feelings that are painful or uncomfortable for the patient, and in developing a sense of safety when the therapist responds nonjudgmentally. The idea of encouraging the expression of thoughts that may not seem socially appropriate or completely relevant to the topic at hand is a cornerstone of psychoanalytic treatments. In a symptom-focused dynamic treatment such as this one, it is used in a particular, adapted fashion, as a guiding principle of dedicated and active exploration rather than as an invitation to long periods of musing or uninterrupted monologue. That is, it is most helpful to let the patient know that exploring even "irrelevant thoughts" can be quite important in understanding how the patient's mind works. However, the therapist will take a very active stance in listening and directing the patient's attention to the potential clues that utterances provide for understanding the patient's depression, rather than listening in a more open-ended fashion for extended periods.

It is also useful to introduce the idea of transference, in some form, early on in the treatment, usually by letting the patient know that one way of investigating troubling or depressing aspects of relationships with others is to see how these may emerge with the therapist and to explore them together. It can be useful to explain that in close relationships with anyone, feelings of confusion or concern about the other person's reactions, or about one's own, are inevitable, and that exploring these confusions may be extremely helpful. (For a useful discussion of working with the transference, see Cooper 1987.) The patient is thus invited to tell the therapist about reactions to what he or she says or does. Finally, the therapist may ask the patient to bring in dreams and notes that responses to films, literature, music, and so on may also be relevant to the therapeutic work.

Sometimes the best method of introducing these concepts is a practical one: rather than encouraging a patient to bring in dreams, the therapist may ask to be told a recent dream. Asking a patient directly, rather than generally, for initial reactions to the therapist can be also helpful.

Case Example 1

After a few introductory sessions with Ms. D, a 40-year-old journalist, during which her childhood in a war-torn country and her current depression were explored, her therapist recommended psychodynamic psychotherapy.

> THERAPIST: It's usually helpful in therapy to discuss your reactions to our work and to me, even if that seems a little rude or awkward. Is there anything you can tell me about that so far?
>
> MS. D [*surprised*]: Well, no, not really... I just... Well, you know I had a consultation with someone else at the same time that we were having our interviews. I really want to find the right therapist. At first, I thought I would go with the other person for sure. She seemed so charismatic. You are quieter. In fact, at first you reminded me of my grandmother, the one I had to stay with when my mother was sick. She was weak, really under my grandfather's thumb. He really frightened me; he had such a bad temper. I never thought she would help me out if he got angry at me. So at first I thought, *No,*

this time I am not getting stuck with my grandma! But then, you said some things that made sense to me. I think you might understand me better. I've never really had that experience before. I always felt like...a Martian or an alien. So I think I will try this out.

Ms. D's therapist had the impression that she never would have heard this significant piece of early transference had she not asked directly for it. This early reaction alerted the therapist to the patient's pressing concerns in the transference about being protected and adequately understood, concerns that would emerge repeatedly in the treatment of this woman's severe mood disturbance.

Introducing the Exploratory Process

Psychodynamic treatment is distinguished from others by its emphasis on gradually deepening investigation of the unconscious motivations, desires, fantasies, and feelings that may determine our moods, beliefs, and even our behaviors. Once a patient is educated about the typical presentation for depression and the nature of psychodynamic treatment, the therapist introduces the concept that people's depressive symptoms *always* have a particular *individual content*. For instance, one patient may be self-critical or guilty about vengeful fantasies, whereas another patient may feel this way about certain sexual wishes. (For a fuller discussion of the concept of unconscious fantasies, see Arlow 1969.) The therapist should explore, from the beginning, what comes to mind for the patient about each prominent symptom and under which situations or circumstances these symptoms might arise. The therapist should also determine the temporal pattern of the patient's internal experiences. For example, the patient may experience intense guilt or self-criticism after mentioning particular fantasies or behaviors. By exploring symptoms and feelings in this manner, the patient begins to understand that the symptoms are meaningful and have particular, understandable origins. This is quite valuable for a patient who feels initially helpless and hopeless about an illness. A more extended case example demonstrating the introduction of dynamic exploration to a patient follows.

Case Example 2

Ms. E was a married accountant in her early 40s when she presented for treatment of a melancholic depression. She was profoundly sad and prominently self-blaming. She accused herself, for instance, of being a terrible patient whom a previous therapist had dismissed as "whining and complaining" all the time.

The therapist decided to evaluate this description further in an attempt to understand the origin of this patient's intense self-criticism. To her great interest, the investigation of this "whining and complaining" revealed a considerable psychological capacity and an important determinant of this patient's depression.

THERAPIST: Can you tell me what he meant by "whining and complaining"?

MS. E [*wryly*]: Oh, it's what they all say! I mean, it's true. I do complain a lot. My mother always told me that.

THERAPIST: When would she say that?

MS. E [*reflecting*]: Well, my sister—she's only a year and a few months older than me. She was just, I think, an easier child for my mother. My mother was young when she had us, 19. When I think about what I was like at 19, no wonder! But of course, I couldn't have seen it that way then. Anyway, my sister just seemed content with things, where I always…I just always wanted more. And I guess I just couldn't shut up about it! [*Laughs but seems simultaneously tearful*]

THERAPIST: What kind of things did you get upset about?

MS. E: Oh, well. My mom was depressed, I think. Or overwhelmed by us, maybe. But I remember her just sleeping a lot. When we went to school—even in kindergarten, it must have been, because I can picture it there in that house—she couldn't really function well in the mornings. I remember my dad waking us up, and then my sister and I would make our lunches. My sister seemed good at it, really, but sometimes I would maybe tear the bread and then get upset about it. I guess I would complain and be a nuisance.

THERAPIST: Do you think maybe that was a lot for your mother to expect, for you to get up at that age and make your own lunch?

MS. E [*surprised*]: Well, maybe. I don't know. I just always felt I couldn't quite do it right. And I'd get upset. And cry. I couldn't help it, really, but it made her so mad and upset with me. [*Sobbing*] You know, I remember one time, after she got so angry. I was sent to my room, and I remember just looking at myself in the mirror, thinking, *What's different about me? What's wrong with me? Why can't I be more like my sister?*

THERAPIST: You felt so bad that you couldn't be the way she wanted you to be. But as you say, she was so young and so

> overwhelmed. Maybe it wasn't so much that *you were over-whelming* as that it was hard for her to manage two very young children at such a young age herself.
>
> MS. E: Well, that may be true. I really have to think about it. But why am I still complaining? People do see me that way, and I don't think they are always wrong...
>
> THERAPIST: That sounds like something for us to explore!

In this case, the early exploration of Ms. E's self-accusation was extremely fruitful. It established that this patient was capable of looking at her mother from different vantage points, using mentalization skills (see subsection "Attachment Theory" in Chapter 2) ("When I think about what I was like at 19, no wonder!"). It also introduced this patient to a way of seeing her depressive symptoms as meaningful. A process began through which she would gain a better understanding of her long-standing feelings of rejection, a key to her narcissistic vulnerability. In this context, Ms. E began to experience hope.

Establishing the Therapeutic Alliance

The term *therapeutic alliance* (Greenson 1967; Stern et al. 1998) refers to the relationship between therapist and patient as they work together in partnership to understand the meaning of the patient's symptoms. As the therapist is seen as caring but dispassionate and dedicated to understanding the meaning of the patient's difficulties without "taking sides" or being judgmental or invasive, a relationship evolves in which the patient learns to trust the therapist with the most intimate fears and sadness. This is crucial because only in the context of a trusting relationship can a patient feel truly comfortable exposing areas of shame and vulnerability in order to do the necessary therapeutic work (see Spezzano 1993; Stone 1981).

Through the therapeutic alliance, patients may also begin to identify with the therapist's way of looking at their difficulties. Optimally, patients learn to incorporate this stance over time into their own repertoire, beginning to inquire, as the therapist might, about the origins and meanings of their symptoms. Through a good working alliance, patients may be helped to overcome their shame about exposing inadequacies or may start to reflect on their excessive guilt.

An awareness of the core dynamics of depression is invaluable in forging a productive alliance with a depressed patient, because this knowledge can guide the therapist from the outset to a deeper exploration of the initial history and of the patient's psychological response to events that triggered the depressive episode. The therapist can best engage the patient's psychological curiosity and help the patient feel understood by keeping these dynamics in mind and using them to make early connections between the patient's painful symptoms and the experience of self and others. For example, in the case of Ms. E, the therapist suggested early developmental origins of her view of herself as complaining that helped her to identify that she might be unfairly self-critical in this regard. With this approach, the therapist is also seen as a dependable and knowledgeable authority on the patient's illness.

Because of the depressed patient's susceptibility to feelings of loss, rejection, and abandonment, many such patients are hungry for a connection that feels solid, responsive, and understanding. This connection alone can provide a powerful motivation for treatment and can in itself help the patient to feel less alone and more hopeful. Because of their fragile self-esteem, such patients also welcome the opportunity to identify with a therapist who seems knowledgeable and assured. Finally, the opportunity to investigate which areas of their self-image are faulty and which are accurate is often welcome as well, because depressed patients can be quite confused about realistically appraising their thoughts, behaviors, and attributes.

Sometimes these sources of motivation backfire and lead to eventual resistances to the interpretive work, a topic that is explored in Chapters 5 ("The Middle Phase of Treatment") and 13 ("Managing Impasses and Negative Reactions to Treatment) of this volume. The term *resistance* is used to mean an obstacle to the progression of treatment, caused either by the fear and avoidance of experiencing or expressing certain feelings or ideas (some in relation to the therapist) or by the patient's substituting another desire in place of the wish to understand symptoms in treatment. The wish for a caring connection, for example, may result in the patient's excessive dependence on the therapist, with the relationship used predominantly to fulfill a wish to be cared for, rather than to further understanding. This was the case with Mr. B in Chapter 1 ("Introduction"). Also, the hunger to idealize can rapidly switch to a devaluation of the therapist when the patient's fantasies are disappointed. These negative feelings can then trigger guilt and a negative reaction to treatment. These possibilities need to be kept in mind and may at times be anticipated openly with the patient as the treatment alliance is being formed (Jacobson 1971). For example, Ms. D, whose case was discussed earlier (see Case Example 1), seemed initially to idealize the enlivening, charismatic traits of her other potential therapist and to be inclined to devalue the quieter stance of the therapist she chose, because the latter reminded her too much of her timid grandmother. It was helpful to point out to this patient that these reactions might emerge again during the treatment and could be explored so that they would not provide a future source of guilt or of resistance. When disruptions in the alliance do occur, understanding and identifying the transference is one way to repair them.

A working knowledge of the dynamics commonly seen in depression may also be used to overcome the initial resistances that such patients sometimes have toward becoming engaged in a psychotherapeutic treatment, as described in the following section.

Identifying Barriers to Engagement in Treatment of Depressed Patients

Excessive Shame and Fear of Exposure

Some depressed patients are initially quite resistant to treatment because of their exquisite susceptibility to shame and their difficulty tolerating an exposure to the therapist of a shameful vulnerability (Kilborne 2002). Managing this difficulty is important from the start, and a sensitive acknowledgement of its existence, paired with an understanding of its role in actually contributing to depression, can be useful in establishing a good initial alliance.

Case Example 3

Mr. F, a 46-year-old businessman, presented with a highly agitated depression, after making a mistake in a new job setting that he feared would result in his being fired. He was in such a state of anxiety that it was difficult for him to even realistically appraise how damaging the error might have been. Mr. F was frank about his distaste for the idea of treatment, including psychotropic medication, from the outset of his first interview: "I avoid this kind of thing at all costs. I always thought all those people on Prozac or going to therapists were unbalanced or felt sorry for themselves or didn't want to accept life as it is. I never, ever imagined that I would be here." Then he outlined, in an embarrassed and rather minimized way, his presenting symptoms of tearfulness, agitation, insomnia, and intense anxiety. He kept obsessively reviewing his mistake, which had involved getting into an argument with a man in a competing department, unnecessarily antagonizing him. This man was now making it impossible for Mr. F to accomplish his first assignment.

As Mr. F realized the consequences of the argument with his adversary, the depression and anxiety he experienced made him feel further out of control and in further jeopardy at work. His sense of shame and exposure led him to attempt to compensate repeatedly in the interview. Mr. F spent a good deal of time assuring the therapist that he was very aware of his mistake, that he was actually very knowledgeable about himself and about his field, and that were he the judging partner, he would likely question his new associate's judgment too.

The therapist realized at that point that it would be essential to address the patient's shame, both as a factor in the dynamics of his depression and as a means to engage him in an alliance in which he felt comfortable exploring these painful issues. She gently encouraged an exploration of his fantasies about the painful episode.

THERAPIST: What do you imagine your new business partners think about you?

MR. F: That I'm cocky. Arrogant. I got into a stupid argument without realizing that I couldn't win. That's bad judgment.

THERAPIST: Have you been viewed as arrogant before?

MR. F: Well, not usually. I've been more concerned I would be seen as too passive, not "take charge" enough. This is really a pretty classy firm. I think I wanted to go in and show them what I could do. But I obviously overdid it.

These initial statements and fantasies prompted certain therapeutic guesses on the part of the clinician treating Mr. F. One obvious thread in the story was his fear of being seen as passive or weak and his preoccupation with instead seeming aggressive and "taking charge." For Mr. F, aggression seemed to imply a manly competence; passivity, a denigrated vulnerability. In his effort not to display denigrated—in this case, passive—parts of his personality, Mr. F became very aggressive. However, he felt he would be punished for the aggression, and this expectation created anxiety and a renewed sense of vulnerability.

The therapist's first task, then, was to tell Mr. F something about her initial understanding of this dynamic in a way that would both be recognizable to him and respect the importance that he placed on others' perceptions of him as knowledgeable and "in charge." Because Mr. F emphasized that coming to treatment felt humiliating, it was particularly important that he experience the process as a mutual encounter in which he could learn more about and master this fear of being seen as inadequate, rather than as a damaging exposure of weakness.

THERAPIST: So you became concerned in this new firm that people see you as in control of things. To accomplish this, as you say, you overdid it. You pushed too hard and alienated this man.

MR. F: Yes.

> THERAPIST: I realize that you don't really like having to come here for help. What you want most is to be back in control of things—especially this depression. But to do that, we really have to understand more about this idea that you're not seen as aggressive or take charge enough, since that's what got you into trouble. You tried way too hard to be seen that way! Have you felt that way before, at other times?

The intervention allowed therapist and patient to identify a central dynamic immediately (that the patient has a particular area of narcissistic vulnerability, his fear of being seen as weak, passive, or, through the lens of his depression, shamefully out of control) and to forge an alliance based on exploration of it. The idea that caused the most trouble for him would be respectfully explored, not as an acknowledgement of inadequacy but as a complex fear contributing to his depression and simultaneously making it difficult for him to seek the help that he needed.

Oppressive, Conscious Guilt and Fear of Its Exacerbation

For other patients, a sense of conscious, oppressive guilt may make therapeutic engagement feel dangerous, as they fear that the treatment will only intensify this self-condemning feeling. Sometimes this can even be expressed as a fear that the therapist will somehow "trick" them into forgiving themselves. These patients may have the unconscious fantasy that their increased competence may be damaging to others (Freud 1916; Klein 1940). Alternatively, they may fear that other fantasies will be revealed in treatment that will trigger further guilt, such as specific sexual or aggressive fantasies. As in the following case example, the therapist can aid this problem by calling attention to the intensity of the patient's guilty feelings and pointing out particular issues that seem to trigger them, questioning the degree of guilt they cause, and exploring alternative underlying reasons for the guilty self-assessment.

Case Example 4A

Ms. G, a journalist in her 30s, initially resisted an exploration of her history and illness because of her fear of discovering something blameworthy.

> Ms. G: I don't think I want to know why I'm depressed. I'm only going to wind up feeling worse about myself.

THERAPIST: Why do you think that?

MS. G: I think that therapists blame parents for everything. Especially mothers. My mom is great—we're very close. She can be totally exasperating, too, of course, but that's human nature. If I learned that deep down, I wanted to hurt her in any way—you know, like the Oedipus complex or something—I think I would just feel so bad I would want to kill myself.

THERAPIST [*after pause*]: You know, I'm not interested in blaming anyone for your depression. I *would* like to understand with you what is contributing to it, though. If we wind up talking about your relationships with people, now or in your earlier life, I would like to help you to understand those in as full and grown-up a way as possible.

In this interchange, the therapist avoided reassuring her guilty patient that she had done nothing wrong, which might only ring untrue or frighten her that her guilty feelings were not being taken seriously. Moreover, such reassurances would do little to advance Ms. G's understanding of herself and her depression. The therapist did emphasize, instead, that therapy was a process through which depression (and conflicted relationships) might be understood. This might signal to the patient that guilt-provoking childhood feelings and fantasies would be understood in a complex manner, not as accurate assessments of the patient's level of responsibility. The therapist recognized that Ms. G's level of fear of blaming her parents was excessive and indicated conflict about negative feelings toward them.

In addition to this preliminary intervention, Ms. G's therapist decided to explore her history for ideas about why she might feel so guilty while explicitly examining her sense of chronic guilt and her fears that this would be exacerbated with treatment. Because the patient mentioned being afraid of what she would discover about her feelings toward her mother, the therapist listened carefully for clues to this guilt as she asked about the childhood history.

THERAPIST: Could you tell me a bit about your earlier life? I would like to learn a little more about the things that might have shaped who you are, how you see things now.

MS. G: Well, it was, you know, a pretty normal childhood. My mom was the stay-at-home–baking cookies sort of mother. We were close.

THERAPIST: And your adolescence?

MS. G: That was harder. When I was 13, Mom was diagnosed with cancer. She was very sick for several years—had radiation therapy, surgery, a lot of procedures. Thank God she recovered.

THERAPIST: That must have been terribly frightening for you.

MS. G: Yes. I really admire her a lot. She pulled through all those awful treatments. It was horrible.

THERAPIST: How was it for you, seeing her go through all of that?

MS. G [*tearfully*]: It was sad! She was so weak and tired. She couldn't do a lot. And my father was pretty overwhelmed. She was in the hospital for a long time at one point.

Noting to herself that Ms. G has a difficult time addressing her own reactions to this devastating event, the therapist nonetheless persists in trying to understand how her patient might have experienced her mother's illness, and especially how this experience might have contributed to her prominent sense of guilt.

THERAPIST: That must have been very hard for you. How did you deal with all of it? Do you remember?

MS. G: My father needed a lot of help. I think I felt more grown-up than the other kids in my class. They never had to deal with anything like that. They wound up seeming sort of immature—kind of clueless—to me.

THERAPIST: So the whole situation created a distance between you and other kids your age. I guess you felt like they couldn't possibly understand what you were going through.

MS. G: Yeah, I felt like either they were from outer space or I was.

THERAPIST: How was it for you at home? You said you helped your father a lot. Did your parents recognize how difficult this was for you?

MS. G: Well, no…[*Begins to cry*] I think my mom was too sick to really register what was going on with me. And my father just wanted me to help. "Do the cleaning. Do the cooking." He couldn't do any of that. I could never feel upset with him, but I did feel frustrated about his asking for so much. I don't think he really thought about how it was for me. And they were having a hard time together, too.

THERAPIST: How so?

MS. G [*sobbing*]: It was awful. My father really isn't the kind of person to be able to handle things like this. My mother, I guess, took care of him emotionally. And for her to not be able to do that…I think he felt bad for her, but I think he also blamed her, in a way. I heard him complaining to her once that all he did was take care of her and got nothing for himself. I was so upset when he said that to her!

The therapist had many guesses about the impact of this history on her patient's tendency to feel guilty. It seemed likely that Ms. G had felt terribly alone during those decisive years in her life, as she was becoming a young woman. Instead of her passage into adulthood being noted or supported, it was overshadowed by the poignant family circumstances. Ms. G might have been upset with her mother, to whom she had been close, for being so un-available when she was ill. She also seemed to have experienced a good deal of disappointment and frustration with her father in those years, which she had tried her best to minimize. Feeling guilty about her angry feelings then, when the family was in crisis and she felt self-indulgent about addressing her own needs, likely contributed to her continued guilt now.

> THERAPIST: You know, it must have been hard for you to be going through all the stuff that teenagers do, at a time when your parents were so upset and preoccupied. Your mother certainly wasn't able to be very available to you then, because she was so sick. And it sounds like you were disappointed in your father and the way he handled things. But you tried really hard not to make a fuss, because of how sick your mother was. Maybe that makes you extra worried about wanting any attention now or about being angry or disappointed with other people.
>
> MS. G [*tearfully*]: You really think that has something to do with why I'm depressed now? I've just been feeling so alone and sad; it feels like I'm going crazy.

These interventions helped Ms. G to overcome her resistance to exploring her depression dynamically. Once she began to feel involved in this process, her therapist continued to focus on understanding her guilty feelings and looking for ways in which they connected to her current depression. This work is discussed further in the section "Clarifying the Central Depressive Psychodynamics" below.

Overvalued Explanations for Depression

Some patients enter treatment with their own explanations of their depression, resulting from defensive attempts to avoid feelings that seem dangerous, shameful, or otherwise intolerable. For example, patients may insist that their mood state is entirely biological, with no psychological determinants at all. Patients who have had a recent loss may invoke that experience as if it entirely explains their current psychological state. To address this view, the therapist must respect patients' dearly held beliefs while broadening the scope of their understanding that various psychological issues may contribute to depression. Ms. H is an example of such a patient.

Case Example 5

A 38-year-old lawyer, Ms. H contacted her therapist 2 weeks after a painful breakup with Tom, her boyfriend of 5 years. Ms. H felt devastated by the breakup, especially because it followed years of unrelenting effort to resolve the issue of Tom's commitment to her. She had made it clear for some time that she wanted to have a child, and she was often infuriated when he told her that he could not consider having a baby for many more years. Finally, Tom had decided to end their relationship in order not to "have this on my conscience."

Ms. H was so upset that she could barely function, wanted only to sleep, and had passive suicidal thoughts: "I wish a car would run over me and put me out of my misery. I really can't bear to imagine my life without children, being one of those lonely women who never has a family. That's worse than death." She spent many of her waking hours ruminating about what had gone wrong. Ms. H vacillated between condemning herself as a pathetic woman who had never been truly loved by Tom and hence was missing some crucial "feminine power," and feeling that Tom was an inhuman man and that she had been unbelievably foolish not to have acted sooner on her concerns about his problematic commitment.

Ms. H had been in a previous dynamic treatment that did not focus specifically on her depression. She felt comfortable with the idea of exploring the meaning of her symptoms; nonetheless, she tended to resist her therapist's initial efforts to identify the meaning of her depression beyond offering teary self-accusations or claiming sadly that it was "obvious why I'm depressed—who wouldn't be, in this situation?" Her therapist decided that it might be most effective to explore this resistance directly, by engaging Ms. H in considering the difference between sadness regarding a significant loss and clinical depression. Although the symptoms the therapist refers to would lead to a consideration of medication, in this instance she is emphasizing the severity of symptoms from the psychological standpoint.

> THERAPIST: You know, I can understand that you would be *really very sad* about this. But you are more than just sad. You can't eat or sleep; you're wishing that you were dead. That's something else entirely. Why do you think that you are depressed right now, rather than simply grieving?
>
> Ms. H [*startled*]: Well, I'm not sure. I have had depressions on and off, since I was an adolescent. Maybe that's part of what drove Tom away. But I can also be really...high-spirited. I know that he loves that part of me. I think that I can be...really a lot of fun and entertaining, and people enjoy that. I enjoy it about myself. I think that maybe people get used to that part of me. Then, when I really need something or want something, maybe they don't take me seriously or get turned off by it. I don't know what to do about that.
>
> THERAPIST: How did this work in your family?
>
> Ms. H: Well, I thought until my last treatment that I had been close to my mom. She could be really fun and caring. But at

other times, she would drift off. My father drank when he got home and would just read the newspaper and get very quiet or angry and moody. I never expected anything much from him. But he was her husband. She just kept trying to engage him. I guess she felt alone, and I'm not really sure how much she really did focus on me—on figuring out who I was.

THERAPIST: It must have been frustrating when she would drift off.

MS. H [*thoughtful*]: It's hard to remember, really. I guess I did try to get her attention back…with my brothers, too. They were older and I just adored them. If I was entertaining, I could get them involved with me.

THERAPIST: Is it still like that with your family?

MS. H: I still am the one who tries to bring everybody together, like for holidays and stuff. Otherwise, I'm afraid everyone would go his own way.

THERAPIST: So it's been your job to entertain your family, to put aside asking directly for what you need, in favor of just being fun to try to get their attention. Was it like that with Tom?

MS. H: In some ways it was. I've known that there were some patterns going on in this relationship, but I haven't been able to do anything about them. Do you think I can ever get over this? I want Tom to marry me! I hope that it's not too late.

THERAPIST: I don't know, but it seems as if this way of trying to be close to someone is really familiar to you. You seem to feel that you have to wrest affection out of the people you love, and that you can never give up.

Ms. H clearly recognized this style of engaging in relationships and seemed intrigued about her difficulty in letting go or in pursuing less frustrating attachments. This curiosity formed the beginnings of an early treatment alliance.

Clarifying the Central Depressive Psychodynamics

Once the therapeutic frame has been established and as the therapeutic alliance begins to form, the therapist helps the patient recognize the unique dynamics central to the depression. A preliminary formulation of these dynamics can aid patients in understanding how this approach may be helpful for their depression, and can thereby strengthen the early therapeutic alliance. For example, with Mr. F, whose case was discussed earlier (see Case Example 3), the therapist concluded that a vulnerability to seeing himself as passive or unmanly had contributed to a compensatory aggressive posturing about which he felt guilty. Further, his aggression had provoked an embarrassingly public retaliation, leaving the patient ashamed and feeling diminished. The guilt, shame, and feelings of inadequacy and self-condemnation that followed seemed to trigger his depression (see depression cycle 1 [Figure 2–1] in Chapter 2, "Development of a Psychodynamic Model of Depression"). As therapist and patient explored this dynamic further, they were able to connect Mr. F's tendency to experience himself as too passive or unmasculine to teasing interactions in his childhood with an athletic brother and with his demanding father about which he still felt quite sensitive. These feelings were identified as triggered in other settings in the past, when Mr. F had also become depressed, seemingly "out of the blue." Working with this material was quite helpful to this patient, as it gave him a sense of predictability and control over his feelings. He began to anticipate when he might feel vulnerable to shameful self-perceptions and to understand and act on these differently.

Mr. F's therapist also explored his tendency to idealize certain men who were in authority positions and, by identifying with them, to feel better about himself. However, this patient would sharply devalue himself if he felt that he had disappointed these men, as had occurred just prior to this depression. Although Mr. F had indeed made a mistake at that time, he was much more devaluing and self-critical than he needed to be, escalating his depressed reaction (see depression cycle 2 [Figure 2–2] in Chapter 2).

With Ms. G, whose case was discussed earlier (see Case Example 4A), an early therapeutic focus that linked her guilty feelings from adolescence to current difficulties with her boyfriend and widespread struggles in adult life with managing angry feelings was decisive in relieving her depressive symptoms.

Case Example 4B

At the time of her presentation for treatment, Ms. G was angry with her boss but unable to confront him. She alternated between castigating herself for being too angry about her work situation and hating herself for "just sitting on all that sense of unfairness and doing nothing about it."

Further, Ms. G was distressed about a growing sense of emotional distance from her boyfriend, who seemed aloof and disengaged from her. She felt sad and lonely as a result but was similarly unable to communicate any of these feelings to him. Her depression combined caustic self-accusations of being a "wimp" for not speaking up about her dissatisfaction at work and with her boyfriend with guilty self-reproaches for being too demanding and difficult. Her therapist attempted to connect these contemporary struggles for Ms. G with her struggles in adolescence and to point out her patient's striking guilt and self-punishment for angry feelings.

> THERAPIST: With your boyfriend being so distant, you feel really alone! I think that makes you upset and disappointed with him, the way you must have been with your father during those years when your mother was so sick and he didn't seem able to recognize the impact of her illness on you at all.
>
> Ms. G: Well, maybe.
>
> THERAPIST: It seems really difficult for you to allow yourself to feel angry with someone, like your father or your boyfriend.
>
> Ms. G [*after long pause*]: My mother is like this, too. When she finally does admit to being angry with my father, she explodes. It all comes out—like too much. Irrational. I'm afraid that's how I'll sound, too, if I ever tried to talk about things. And I hate being angry. I mean, my father and my boyfriend—I kind of understand why they are that way. It seems petty not to be able to get past it.
>
> THERAPIST: But if you let the angry feelings pile up, the way your mother did, if you ignore them instead of acknowledging them, they don't just go away. I think that happens to you at work, too.

In this way, the patient's particular vulnerability to feeling sad or alone when important others became distant, her intense guilt about feelings of frustration or disappointment with others, her avoidance of "irrational, explosive" anger, and her self-accusations of being "wimpy" are connected to meaningful events in her childhood. Her feared identification with her mother's anger as a source of her depression is a common dynamic in depression (see the case of Ms. C in Chapter 2) (Jacobson 1971). This work was quite helpful in diminishing this patient's depressive symptoms in the early treatment phase. More work was required in the middle phase to consolidate this gain, however, and to prevent future episodes, as is seen in Chapter 6 ("Addressing Narcissistic Vulnerability").

Role of Psychoeducation in the Early Treatment Phase

Dynamic therapists educate their patients about the biopsychosocial dimensions of depression throughout their treatment. This is a necessary aspect of any treatment endeavor, in that it encourages patients to take an active role in understanding and managing their illness. Further, it can help particularly during the early treatment phase, when depressed patients may struggle with their sense of shame and exposure. Mr. F was helped to engage in his treatment by a brief explanation of the biological origins of his depression. He was particularly attentive to the explanation that this illness is often comorbid not only with anxiety but also with migraine headaches, which he experienced. This pairing of a painful psychological state with a somatic symptom proved to be face saving for this patient, an indication that he was not "deeply psychologically disturbed."

Establishing the distinction between depression and sadness, which helped Ms. H better focus on understanding her reactions to her loss, is also useful for our patients for other reasons. Accomplished early in treatment, it may help them to see themselves as having a distinct syndrome rather than as being needy or weak. Later, it may provide encouragement for patients to tackle an exploration of painful events in their lives and to distinguish the pain and sadness stirred up in the process from the feared recurrence of an actual depressive episode.

For Ms. G, learning more about what usually happens developmentally during adolescence, in terms of a teenager's struggle for distance from her parents and for a critical, more objective viewpoint toward them, was very helpful. She had regarded these desires, in the context of her mother's illness, as traitorous and self-indulgent and had felt quite guilty about them.

Although the psychoeducation is not formal or didactic, the psychodynamic therapist helps patients to recognize that symptoms have meaning, that developmental factors affect current mental life and relationships, that feelings and fantasies that may be out of awareness can create conflict, and that feelings about the therapist can play a valuable role in learning about these conflicts. The therapist indirectly educates the patient about how these factors contribute to depressive symptoms.

References

Arlow JA: Unconscious fantasy and disturbances of conscious experience. Psychoanal Q 38(1):1–27, 1969 5764146
Cooper AM: Changes in psychoanalytic ideas: transference interpretation. J Am Psychoanal Assoc 35(1):77–98, 1987 3584822
Dewald P: The psychoanalytic psychotherapies, in Textbook of Psychoanalysis. Edited by Nersessian E, Kopff RG Jr. Washington, DC, American Psychiatric Press, 1996, pp 455–484

Freud S: Some character-types met with in psychoanalytic work (1916), in The Standard Edition of the Complete Psychological Works of Sigmund Freud, Vol 14. Translated and edited by Strachey J. London, Hogarth Press, 1957, pp 316–331

Greenson RR: The Technique and Practice of Psychoanalysis. New York, International Universities Press, 1967

Jacobson E: Depression: Comparative Studies of Normal, Neurotic, and Psychotic Conditions. New York, International Universities Press, 1971

Kilborne B: Disappearing Persons: Shame and Appearance. Albany, State University of New York Press, 2002

Klein M: Mourning and its relation to manic-depressive states. Int J Psychoanal 21:125–153, 1940

Kris A: Free Associations: Method and Process. New Haven, CT, Yale University Press, 1962

Meissner WW: Freud and Psychoanalysis. Notre Dame, IN, University of Notre Dame Press, 2000

Spezzano C: Affect in Psychoanalysis: A Clinical Synthesis. Hillsdale, NJ, Analytic Press, 1993

Stern DN, Sander LW, Nahum JP, et al; The Process of Change Study Group: Non-interpretive mechanisms in psychoanalytic therapy. The 'something more' than interpretation. Int J Psychoanal 79(Pt 5):903–921, 1998 9871830

Stone L: Notes on the non-interpretive elements in the psychoanalytic situation and process (1981), in Transference and Its Context. New York, Jason Aronson, 1984, pp 153–176

The Middle Phase
of Treatment

IN the initial phase of depression-focused psychodynamic psychotherapy, the patient's symptoms begin to recede with the development of a hopeful, affectively connected treatment relationship and the beginnings of an understanding that depressive symptoms have meaning. The early, central formulations create a sense of being understood by the therapist, with whose stance toward the depression the patient begins to identify. The patient sees that the depressive symptoms are connected to current and past experience, and hence the symptoms feel less "out of the blue" and more within his or her control.

The patient and therapist now identify their work together as based not only on relieving depressive symptoms but also on reducing the vulnerability to future depressive episodes by increased understanding of their underpinnings and context, aiding in anticipatory control (Table 5–1). They begin to work more extensively with the dynamics already identified, refining and extending an understanding of how the conflicted feelings and fantasies emerged with significant others in the past and present. They examine in depth the presence of the dynamics in various forms—in dreams, fantasies, behaviors, and relationships—paying attention to expression of these dynamics in the transference. The active exploration of feelings with the therapist as they occur often has an immediacy and an affective charge that makes such realizations vital sources of insight. A patient also has the opportunity with the therapist to experiment with different ways of feeling and relating that have seemed forbidden or too risky in the past. This knowledge and the shifts in relating to others can aid in the change of problematic patterns in interpersonal relationships.

Working With the Central Themes

Chapters 6–10 focus in depth on how to explore the major dynamic themes of vulnerability in self-esteem, reactive anger, guilt and self-punishment, tendencies toward idealization and devaluation, and characteristic defenses in depressed patients. In this chapter, we review the basic techniques used in this treatment. These techniques are used in every phase of treatment but constitute the primary work of the important middle phase.

Techniques Used in the Middle Phase

Clarification

The term *clarification* refers to a technique in which patients' typical methods of thinking or feeling about themselves or others are pointed out, in this context particularly as they relate to the depressive mood state (Stone 1981). Similar to interventions in cognitive-behavioral therapy, clarifications do not address patients' unconscious motivations or early contributions to their way of thinking about themselves. Rather, they are used to bring attention to certain self-defeating thought or behavior patterns or to question a characteristic mode of perception that reinforces the depressive mind-set. Once this is brought to patients' attention, a period of exploration and further clarification eventually leads to an interpretation. An example of a clarification follows.

Case Example 1

Ms. I, a graduate student who was almost 30 years old and had just recovered from a major depression, brought in the following dilemma to her therapist: She was foundering in her work on a long paper for an important course toward the end of her last semester in her master's program. She found herself unfocused and having difficulty getting to the library to do needed research. At the same time, she was planning to throw herself a thirtieth birthday party. But work on the paper was detracting from time she needed to spend on the party, and Ms. I was despairing that neither would be successful. "So, I want a real celebration of all my friends who stuck with me when I was so depressed. I want to show everyone that de-

---

Table 5–1.   Middle phase of depression-focused dynamic psychotherapy

---

Aim: reducing vulnerability to further episodes

1. Review, clarification, and expansion of central themes and their contributions to depressive mind states
2. Strengthening the therapeutic alliance; further work with the transference
3. Recognizing how the underlying dynamics lead to problematic patterns in interpersonal relationships, allowing for changes in these patterns

Techniques

1. Clarification
2. Confrontation
3. Interpretation: defense, genetic, conflict, superego
4. Interpretation of the transference
5. Attention paid to the countertransference
6. Interpretation of dreams, slips of the tongue, etc.

---

pression isn't all of me: I can also have a lot of fun! But if I work hard on the party, then I feel like a frivolous person who can't be serious. And if I work on the paper, I think that I'm dull and will never have a life outside of academics! My party will fall flat because I didn't spend enough time planning it and I will feel like a failure!"

Her therapist, who had learned that Ms. I responded well to humor, pointed out that in fact, she was becoming an expert at making herself miserable! She was regarding the different goals that she had for herself (to be both a successful academic and a happy, involved friend) as competing with each other, when there was no evidence that they had to be. When she imagined that these were mutually exclusive, she could then torment herself by assuming that she would attain neither one, because she wanted each goal too much to forsake the other. This clarification helped Ms. I to reevaluate her beliefs and to explore why she felt her goals were contradictory and self-expectations so extreme.

Confrontation

This technique, a special kind of clarification, conveys a thoughtful, empathic, but strongly worded statement about a patient's self-destructive or aggressive behavior or a contradictory set of perceptions that makes depression more likely. It is often used when the patient seems to have a stake in ignoring what has been learned in the therapeutic work, and it carries an emotional impact that can significantly affect treatment (Stone 1981). Phrases often used to point out such behaviors include "Have you noticed that you are…?"

and "It may have slipped by you, but each time I have suggested *x*, you have tended to…"

Case Example 2

Mr. J, a 50-year-old lawyer, was chronically anxious and depressed and had recently recovered from a severe episode of major depression. Any sense of relief he obtained from the subsiding of his depressive symptoms, however, seemed to rapidly vanish as he became preoccupied by somatic complaints. He insisted that he was beset by angina, despite multiple, extensive negative cardiac workups, and could not seem to stop voicing these concerns. He seemed upset with his cardiologist, despite the fact that this doctor had taken his complaints very seriously. His therapist was concerned that the patient was alienating this helpful physician, to his own detriment, and was ignoring insights he had gained earlier in their treatment. The therapist finally voiced his conclusion that Mr. J seemed bent on seeing himself as quite ill, whether from depression or from heart disease, even though he had substantially recovered from the more severe symptoms of his depression and had negative findings on his cardiac workup.

> THERAPIST: You know, many people would be relieved to be given a clean bill of health! You seem to be having a really hard time feeling *any* relief about it, though, and I am afraid that you may be pushing away those who have been trying hard to help out. Maybe it is *very*, very hard for you to see yourself as *not* being sick or in need of a lot of care. I think you are afraid that others won't give you what you really need from them. I know that was your experience with your parents, and I know how hard that was for you! But it just might not be true of every person in your life whom you need help from now!

This strong but empathically expressed statement startled the patient and led to a heartfelt discussion of his sense of loneliness as a child when he felt sad or distressed. He often had experienced these feelings as belittled or even derided by his family. Physical complaints were sometimes seen as more acceptable, gaining him attention and care, though this was rather erratic and hard to count on. This example also suggests how patients may push away others because of an expectation that they will not be responsive, adding to their sense of aloneness.

Interpretation

Interpretation adds another dimension to the kinds of interventions noted above. Interpretations tie observed behaviors or thought patterns to the dynamic factors that may give rise to them, and they usually follow a period of exploration, during which the therapist develops a hypothesis about the underpinnings of the patient's symptoms. Interpretive probes are often offered in the form of a question by the therapist, to open up avenues of potentially fruitful investigation. As noted previously, an interpretation as part of an early formulation can provide an initial scaffolding for understanding contributors to the patient's depression. Further interpretations are made when the therapist judges that they will be convincing and easily seen to connect with previously discussed, familiar conflicts. Interpretations thus proceed stepwise throughout a treatment, building on one another so that they accrue an increasing power to explain myriad interrelated symptoms and behavioral patterns. A patient's response to an interpretation can add to its relevance and completeness.

There are a limited number of types of interpretation, based on the nature of the clinical material addressed. Defense interpretations, discussed at length at in Chapter 10 ("Defense Mechanisms in Depressed Patients"), consider the ways in which patients characteristically defend themselves from painful affects and perceptions of themselves and others, or threatening unconscious fantasies. A defense interpretation might point out to a patient how difficult he finds it to be angry and how he defends against this strong feeling by continually substituting a resolute cheeriness when in fact he is quite upset (a form of reaction formation). Although this defense may serve to deflect others' anger toward the patient, it makes it difficult for them to really understand him, depriving the patient of the experience of emotional closeness that he may crave. This is another example of how problematic intrapsychic conflicts can adversely affect interpersonal relationships.

Genetic (referring to origins or genesis rather than heredity) interpretations tie in past experiences, perceptions, or fantasies with current thoughts or behavior. For example, Ms. D, whose case was first mentioned in Chapter 4 ("Getting Started With Psychodynamic Treatment of Depression"; see Case Example 1), was the immigrant from a war-torn country who was sent to live with her grandparents. Her treatment unearthed Ms. D's vivid feelings of helplessness and fear due to this separation from her parents. She felt that she had to always be on her best behavior in order to be worthy of getting her mother back, and she was frightened by angry, disloyal thoughts she had about her mother during her absence. In the present, Ms. D despaired about her difficulty communicating with her husband when she felt disappointed with him. She was afraid that her anger would cause him to leave her, but she could not bear the distance she felt from him when she could not articulate her feelings. Ms. D was helped considerably by genetic interpretations linking her current fears with this powerful past experience. Understanding the origin of her difficulty made it somewhat easier for her to begin to communicate with her husband.

Other kinds of interpretations highlight unconscious wishes or conflicts that the patient seems to have, or address elements of the superego.

Interpretations of the Transference

Although defense, genetic, conflict, and superego interpretations are used in every phase of treatment, transference interpretations are used most widely in the middle and termination phases. Interpreting the transference at this time, when the therapeutic alliance is established and patients may feel more comfortable looking at their relationship with the therapist, enables them to understand characteristic ways in which they may misperceive or act in a self-defeating manner with others. In fact, the greatest attention in treatment is usually paid to transference manifestations that seem to generalize to other important relationships in patients' lives (see Cooper 1987; Westen and Gabbard 2002). When patients can learn about those characteristic feelings and behaviors toward the therapist that also recur with others to whom they are attached, who may frustrate them or be perceived as wielding authority, for example, they develop a much greater awareness of the motivations for their actions and experiences. This can aid in a shift in their management of their relationships with others.

For depressed patients, common misperceptions involve a sense that others judge them, find them inadequate, or will be inevitably disappointing and frustrating, especially in their caretaking capacity. Common enactments (acting on such ideas in the treatment) can involve subtle or frank invitations to the therapist to participate with the individual in a sense of victimization or to become involved in mutual, unrealistic idealization or devaluation. (For a more extensive discussion of this topic, see Rothstein et al. 1999.)

One opportunity for transference interpretation occurs when an otherwise evolving therapeutic alliance seems to become disrupted (Safran and Muran 2000). For example, Ms. K, a 35-year-old architect who had been speaking freely and volunteering her reflections on her symptoms, came into session one day sullen and self-berating. When her therapist asked her what she thought might be wrong, the patient sniped.

Case Example 3

Ms. K: I guess I'm depressed. That's what I'm here for, right?

THERAPIST: Yes, and you often have ideas about what might be happening.

Ms. K: Well, all that doesn't seem to be getting anywhere, does it?

THERAPIST: You seem upset and angry at yourself, but I have a feeling that you may also be upset with me.

Ms. K: No, of course not. I just feel as if I'm not getting anywhere, and that makes me upset. I had been feeling so good for a while, and this is really demoralizing. Maybe I can't really get much better.

THERAPIST: It seems as if you must be disappointed in me and in your treatment, if you feel that you're stuck feeling badly, with no hope of getting much better.

Ms. K: I guess I'm disappointed, but mostly in myself. Maybe therapy is just another thing that I'm not good at.

THERAPIST: You actually have been very engaged in therapy and talking about things pretty freely here. And you have been doing a lot better. When did you start to feel like this?

Ms. K: When I spoke to my mother on the phone last night. Even with all the things we've understood, it still hurt me when I tried to tell her about my life and she didn't seem to want to listen.

THERAPIST: What happened in the phone call?

Ms. K: I told her about the difficulties I was having at work, and she got freaked out, saying "You need that job!" She blamed me for everything and didn't want to hear my side of things. That's how it often felt with her. I got really upset.

THERAPIST: I can see how hurt you feel, and also how disappointed and angry you are with her. You turn your anger against *yourself*, though, when you claim that *you're* the disappointment who's no good at therapy. It's as if you were saying, "All right, Mom, you're blaming me; I may as well join in and blame myself, too." You're punishing yourself for feeling hurt and vulnerable and angry, and *indirectly*, you are also punishing me. How good could *I* be if I'm not helping you feel less vulnerable and angry at her? And how good a mother can *she* be, if you get off the phone feeling so hurt?

Ms. K: I know that's not realistic, but it is how I was feeling about things.

Here, the patient's turning her anger inward is highlighted, as well as the fact that her self-punishment is also indirectly an indictment of both mother and therapist. In the transference, the patient's disappointment and blaming extends to her therapist, experienced and treated as another disappointing maternal figure who does not adequately protect her. This vignette also demonstrates how a surge in symptoms occurs in a particular context and indicates how patients can steadily learn to examine what is occurring when symptoms worsen. In addition, it shows how patients can come to acknowledge feelings with the therapist, such as anger, which they tend to keep out of awareness. Finally, it demonstrates how patients' anger can be turned inward out of conflict, fueling the severity of the superego (depression cycle 1). Identifying and accepting this anger can help to relieve this process.

As the patient's symptoms and relationships are extensively explored, work in the transference can reveal significant information and provide an important therapeutic tool. Whenever the therapeutic work bogs down, it is helpful to think of what might be happening in the transference—that is, in the patient's conceptualization of the therapist within the working relationship. Of course, transference interpretations may be made at any point in this phase of treatment when they seem to be pertinent and helpful, not only when there appears to be a temporary impasse. In the following case, the therapist makes a series of interpretations that identify several intersecting components of the patient's dynamics.

Case Example 4

Dr. L was a married surgeon in his 40s with two children who was referred for psychotherapy for recurrent, moderately severe depressive episodes. Although he was a man who loved feeling decisive and strong, his therapy had revealed considerable self-hatred whenever he felt as if he were behaving in a "weak" or indecisive fashion. At times, he was also contemptuous of his wife, when he saw her as passive or confused about something. This caused turmoil in their marriage, and his critical outbursts were inevitably followed by self-punishing behavior and by a tormenting sense of guilt.

In the transference, his therapist noted that Dr. L became contemptuous of her and disinclined to work at his treatment when he was actually feeling vulnerable himself. Their exploration of his contempt helped to illuminate his marital difficulties considerably.

> DR. L: I usually pride myself on making decisions with patients easily. I love that about surgery. The decision-making process is so clear, and when there's a judgment call, I'm confident in my judgment. After I went to Boston last month to learn that new procedure, though, I was excited about trying it out, but I got into difficulty with my first patient. The case

went okay in the end, but I'm concerned that I tried this before I was ready. Also, I think the residents noticed my anxiety. I hate that. I don't want them to see me as wishy-washy.

THERAPIST: Can you tell me more about that?

DR. L [*raising his voice*]: What more could you possibly want to hear? People in your field are unbelievable! Do you have to talk about everything? I think it's pretty clear what I was saying! What do *you* think about it?

THERAPIST: I think that we need to understand what got you so upset just now! Why do you think you got so angry about my question?

DR. L: Because I'm impatient with dithering, that's why.

THERAPIST: Look, for some reason, my question provoked a lot of contempt on your part. I'd like to look at that. You said that you felt bad that the residents might think you were wishy-washy. What's that all about? Why is feeling nervous when a procedure is going badly "wishy-washy"?

DR. L [*silent and thoughtful for several minutes*]: Okay, you have a point, I guess. I don't know what got me so riled up. This is exactly the kind of thing that goes on with my wife, when I get so angry with her. The "wishy-washy" thing: I think it has to do with what we've been talking about as "weakness." Being ruffled when I'm doing my job *is* weak. I'm *very* concerned about my reputation. This field is really competitive; if word gets out that I'm nervous or indecisive, I'm sunk! There are, believe me, younger, hungrier men, very aggressive men, just waiting to take over my place.

THERAPIST: And you feel that you have to be very strong to keep them from attacking you and taking over. You know, I wonder if that doesn't have something to do with feeling the need to attack *me* just now.

DR. L: What do you mean?

THERAPIST: You were trying to tell me about what it was like for you in the OR, feeling anxious, which you interpret as being weak. When I asked to hear more, it was very uncomfortable for you. You don't like anyone seeing you that way, and you didn't want to have to talk more and feel more about it! So *you attacked me instead.* In your eyes, *I* become the weak, foolish one, the one who is dithering and not knowing how to do this right. *You* become the masculine, critical person, the one who is able to take over. For that instant, you can stop worrying about feeling weak or about to be attacked: You've just proven how masculine and on top of things you are.

DR. L: I do see what you mean. I guess that you're right. I also think this *does* have something to do with my wife and me.

> Sometimes I see her as very weak, when she's just having a hard time at something. It feels like if *she's* weak, and we're a team, then it reflects on me, too. I hate that!
>
> THERAPIST: So you attack her to prove to the world that it's *not you* who are the weak or passive one or the one having trouble.
>
> DR. L: Yes, I'm afraid so. [*Pauses*] I used to get like that with my mother. She was in a fog a lot of the time. I didn't realize that she had probably been drinking and that because of that, she just *couldn't* pay attention. I would get so furious with her.

In addition to use of the transference, this vignette also provides an example of identifying a pattern of conflicts in various contexts. This helps the patient to develop conviction about the pattern and aids in the process of working through.

At this point, rather than explore the angry feelings further, which the patient was acknowledging, the therapist chose to focus on the sense of vulnerability that the patient must have experienced when his mother was so unavailable. It is this vulnerability, and related affects of sadness, rejection, and confusion, that results in the patient's sense of weakness, his self-hatred, and his turning of this self-condemnation toward others. Rather than ask Dr. L, who was so prone to externalizing or denying his feelings, if he were sad or upset when mother was drinking, the therapist made a point that it must have been so.

> THERAPIST: It must have been frightening when she was so unresponsive.
>
> DR. L: Yes, I think so. Especially because when she wasn't so drunk, she was such a vibrant person!
>
> THERAPIST: And you often see your wife as so vibrant and connected! Except when she is having trouble.
>
> DR. L: Yes. I think that's why I must get so angry when she seems out of it, like she's not getting something. Maybe it brings this up about my mother. She would just seem to…vanish sometimes, like she couldn't see or grasp what I wanted. I hated that.
>
> THERAPIST: It must have made you feel so alone.
>
> DR. L: I suppose so. I don't really let myself remember that.
>
> THERAPIST: Maybe those feelings—of having been sad and so alone sometimes—are part of this idea that you have about yourself as being weak.

Identifying these precipitants for Dr. L's ready rage at disappointing female caretakers was crucial for his treatment. He began to examine his outbursts in a considerably more reflective manner, and gradually, with continued work over many similar episodes, to understand and control them. He became able to differentiate his wife's periods of uncertainty from his mother's more significant problems with alcoholism. As a result, his relationship with his wife was no longer a source of turmoil and guilt, another example of how an understanding of dynamics and work in the transference can positively affect other relationships. The material that was uncovered during this exchange also lead to a deeper appreciation of the sources of his vulnerability.

Later in the treatment with Dr. L, work in the transference illuminated aspects of his deep fear of attack by competitive men. These fears often led Dr. L to behave very aggressively in his own defense, prompting guilt on his part. They continued to contribute to an embarrassed perception of himself as weak and to self-hatred that was diminishing in intensity but still quite real.

> DR. L: I think I missed you when you were away on vacation. I felt there were things we might have talked about. [*Pauses*] I have this idea, as I'm saying this, that you will sense an advantage and leap on it—you will jump on me in some way—because I was…missing you.
>
> THERAPIST: That sounds like the feeling you get at work sometimes, that the other doctors will jump in and take advantage if they sense that you are weak.
>
> DR. L: Yes, I know. It feels like I am expecting you to be like them—critical, competitive, cutthroat—rather than the way I usually see you.
>
> THERAPIST: Critical and cutthroat. Sounds like what we were talking about, before my vacation, about you and your brother.
>
> DR. L: Oh, yes. Only in that relationship, *I* am the attacking one, the younger, less vulnerable one.
>
> THERAPIST: Yes, indeed. You always felt angry that he was older and bigger but that he didn't defend himself from you.

This vignette demonstrates how the patient is beginning to recognize more of the transferential experience in his therapy. In the treatment recently, the patient had been struggling with guilty feelings about having succeeded in his life to a much greater degree than had his older brother. He was angry but also felt quite guilty that his brother had passively allowed him to win at their childhood fights and games.

> DR. L: So you think that I am guilty about all that and that I imagine that you or someone else will do it back to me. Sort of a punishment. I see your point. I think, too, that when I am feeling vulnerable, that I'm being like him—weak. I know

> all too well that someone else may come along and take ad-
> vantage of that. I certainly took advantage of his passivity,
> and I hated him for letting me do it.

This contribution to Dr. L's fears of attack seemed to frequently emerge within the transference. The vignette offers an example of a transference manifestation in which the female therapist is perceived as having qualities similar to that of the male patient himself in relation to his brother, qualities that he feared in other men. This is actually quite common: transference is not limited by gender. Thus, maternal transferences can be experienced with male therapists and paternal transferences with women, and so on, and should be actively looked for.

Yet another contribution to Dr. L's fears of attack, with subsequent depressive affects, emerged in the exploration of a different kind of transference manifestation, still later in the treatment. Dr. L, who gradually became quite attached to his therapist, had been talking about his esteem for her in recent sessions. In the past, his therapist had seen his affection as sometimes romantically, sometimes maternally tinged. In the recent sessions, however, the physician had been speaking of his admiration for her insights, which he described as "sharp" and "incisive." He wanted to discuss decisions that he needed to make, and the therapist had the impression that these conversations were experienced by Dr. L as "man-to-man" rather than as flirtatious or seeking of maternal care. After a number of such sessions, however, Dr. L seemed uncharacteristically quiet and diffident, even slightly depressed.

> THERAPIST: You seem more quiet today, more down than usual.
> DR. L: I was thinking about my department chair last night. I am
> worried that he and these other surgeons, more experienced
> men whom I look up to, will think I am weak, because I ad-
> mire them so much. I actually try to…not hide it, but not
> make a big deal of it.
> THERAPIST: How do you think they might react?
> DR. L: Oh, you know. "Dr. L is losing it! Go in for the kill!"
> THERAPIST: It sounds as if you think they wouldn't *want* your ad-
> miration, that they'd pull away and go on the attack. That's
> kind of a peculiar response, isn't it? I was under the impression
> that people like to be admired!

In this context the therapist is using a mentalization approach, helping the patient to consider what might be going on in the minds of others. The patient then applies this approach in thinking about what motivated his father.

DR. L: Well, except for my father, as you know. I wanted *so* much to have a connection with him, and he had no patience for it. He just couldn't seem to "get" children. And then he died just as I was beginning to get to know him as an adult.

THERAPIST: You feel that other men whom you respect will also pull away or criticize or attack you if they know that deep down, you want to connect with them, talk with them, be with them, as you wanted to be with your father.

DR. L: Yes, I suppose so.

THERAPIST: Might this have something to do with how down and quiet you seem today? I'd gotten the feeling that you've enjoyed talking with me lately, in the way that maybe you wished you could have spoken with your father.

DR. L: Yes. I do wonder if you'll find me "too much" and just decide "that's it—we're done."

THERAPIST: And then you would lose me, just as you lost your father the minute you started feeling you might get comfortable with him.

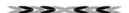

These vignettes demonstrate the value of interpreting transference phenomena connected with conflicts that contribute to the patient's depression. They also demonstrate the evolution of the therapeutic process. Conflicts leading to a depressive diathesis often are multidetermined. For example, Dr. L's sense of vulnerability to attack and his resulting self-hatred related to conflicts about his relationships with his mother, father, and brother. They involved fears of attack for "weakness" as well as distress surrounding others being unresponsive. During the middle phase of treatment, each of these conflicts appeared within the transference, as well as in real-time conflicts with others. The opportunity to work through each of these conflicts helped to significantly reinforce this patient's understanding of himself and of his susceptibility to depression.

The next vignette further demonstrates how a series of conflicts can be worked through in the transference.

Case Example 5

Mr. M was a lawyer in his late 30s with dysthymia and panic disorder; his mother died of cancer when he was an adolescent. His guilt over aggressive and competitive thoughts toward each of his parents was the focal point of much of his treatment. Mr. M imagined that his angry resentment over his mother's controlling behavior had caused her death and was also chronically afraid that he could devastate his father, whom he saw as rather weak.

Mr. M's fears of his aggressive or competitive responses to his therapist were explored at length during the early and middle phases of his treatment. An additional, powerful focus for transference work was provided during the middle phase when Mr. M began to hesitantly discuss emerging sexual feelings for his therapist.

These feelings were first signaled when Mr. M made a slip, referring to "going with" his therapist. When she pointed out that *going with* usually referred to dating, he blushed and acknowledged that the slip was meaningful. He *had* become aware of new, rather romantic feelings for her.

In the treatment at that point, Mr. M had just acknowledged that because he felt less depressed and anxious, his previously stagnant sex life with his wife was improving. Nonetheless, he found it difficult to allow himself to be happy. For instance, he had bought a new, expensive car and taken it for a drive in the country one day, feeling proud and elated. His pleasure was wrecked as he began to speed, misjudged a curve, and drove off the road, incurring some damage to the shiny new vehicle. In examining this, Mr. M associated to fantasies of bodily injury and recalled that starting at age 13, he feared that something terrible would happen to his penis if he became too sexually excited. It became clear to therapist and patient that his damaging the car was a self-punishment exacted from guilt over his recent expansiveness and excitement: buying and enjoying the automobile and enjoying renewed sexual intimacy with his wife. This formulation is consistent with that suggested by Brenner (1979) (see Chapter 2, "Development of a Psychodynamic Model of Depression"), in which patients unconsciously disempower themselves as punishment for what is experienced as conflicted competitive aggressive or sexual wishes.

Now, as he admitted to becoming aware of fond feelings about his therapist, they explored his guilty reactions further. Mr. M recalled that he had been aware of unwanted sexual feelings about his mother prior to her death. He remembered a barely conscious fantasy that her body was being "cut up" (in disfiguring surgeries for the cancer) as a savage punishment for his sexual awareness of her.

Talking about these feelings and having them understood, though difficult, was enormously relieving to Mr. M. He became freer in discussing sexual fantasies, though at times he seemed to do this with the intent of shocking or irking his therapist. She noted that he seemed to feel during these times like a rebellious boy in the transference, as a way of enjoying their connection without having to experience what seemed the threatening aspects of being an adult with her. This was in contrast to other times when Mr. M discussed his sexuality and his transference feelings in a more heartfelt or adult way. As Mr. M contemplated her words, he said sadly, "But if I become an adult, then our therapy is over."

This was a particularly poignant moment for him, as becoming an adult had been inextricably intertwined in reality with losing his mother forever. It allowed Mr. M to vividly understand that enjoying his life in an adult manner was frightening, not only because of his fears of the aggression or competitiveness that he imagined this entailed but also because he deeply feared being left all alone. The guilt that he experienced over his sexuality, and his fears that being an adult meant being abandoned, provided a significant focus for the middle part of his treatment. Without the experience of these feelings within the transference relationship, it is unlikely that Mr. M would have had such a vivid or decisive understanding of his significant inhibitions. These inhibitions, in turn, contributed to his chronic sense of inadequacy as a man, and thus to his dysthymia, which had receded when the treatment ended.

Working With Countertransference Feelings

The many strong affects experienced and directed toward the therapist provoke numerous reactions on the clinician's part. These countertransference reactions were initially thought to interfere with treatment. However, it was soon recognized that they could provide the therapist with a valuable resource for reflection about the meanings of interactions with patients (Gabbard 1995; Jacobs 1993; Makari and Shapiro 1993; Sandler 1976; Shapiro 2002). For example, Dr. L's contemptuous attacks often left his therapist feeling hurt, inadequate, and disempowered. These feelings, so similar to the sense of "weakness" that frightened this patient, helped the therapist to understand the experience that he was working so hard to avoid and was perceiving in her and his wife instead. This understanding, in turn, helped her to feel less personally hurt and significantly more empathic about what her patient was likely experiencing. Similarly, when she became aware of sexual fantasies about Dr. L, the realization helped her to discern his subtle flirtatious behaviors and a gradually emerging romantic transference to which she was responding. (For a more detailed discussion about recognizing and working with such countertransferential feelings, see Gabbard 1994.)

The treatment of Dr. L and the following clinical example demonstrate a crucial aspect of dynamic psychotherapy. Clinicians should always scan their feelings and reactions to patients, because they are often the first sign of significant and meaningful transference. Once clinicians become aware of these feelings, they should carefully consider the clinical material for signs that they are tuning into an aspect of patients' experiences. It is important, however, to be able to distinguish this from therapists' *own*, more generic reactions to certain interpersonal experiences that may provoke affective responses more related to their own dynamics than to those of patients (Gabbard 1995; Searles 1959). In addition, Sandler (1976) offered a term—*role responsiveness*—for situations in which "the irrational response of the analyst, which his professional conscience leads him to see entirely as a blind spot of his own, may sometimes be usefully regarded as a compromise formation between his own tendencies and his reflexive acceptance of the role which the patient is forcing on him" (p. 45). It is for help in distinguishing all these responses that it is often recommended that dynamic therapists have their own treatment at some point in their training.

Case Example 6

Ms. N was a graphic artist in her late 20s who presented with concurrent diagnoses of borderline personality disorder and severe depression. This patient had a history of alcohol abuse and a prior suicide attempt, and her interpersonal relationships were quite stormy. Ms. N would feel upset and victimized if friends or coworkers seemed uncaring and would confront them with tearful, angry recriminations. She paid such attention to the subtle details of her interactions that one former boyfriend chided her that "being in a relationship with you is like reading a book and having to study every footnote."

Her therapist was also quite aware of this, as Ms. N would closely scrutinize every aspect of the clinician's words or behavior for clues about whether she was fully understood. The therapist found herself becoming extremely watchful of her behavior and phrasing, feeling oppressed and resentful, and sympathizing more and more with Ms. N's coworkers. When she realized one day that she was subtly "siding" with these others, rather than attempting to fully understand her patient's behavior, the therapist considered the clinical material to better understand her reactions.

Ms. N had been physically abused by her father, who beat her with a belt for minor infractions of his many rules and regulations. The therapist gradually realized that Ms. N herself must have felt that her every behavior was scrutinized. If she displeased her father, she would be beaten and become terrified and silently, helplessly enraged. The therapist came to understand that Ms. N had learned to closely scrutinize her own behavior and that of others out of a need to gain some control in her relationship with this frightening man, and began to feel much more empathy for her.

> Ms. N: I was really upset with you yesterday, when you said that maybe Jane was finding me "intense." What do you mean by that, anyway? I think that focusing on my relationships is a strength of mine!

THERAPIST: I can understand your confusion. What I was referring to was your tendency to so carefully consider each aspect of your interactions with her. As I've been thinking about it, I realize how much you must have felt that you had to watch *everything* you did with your father. If you didn't, he'd explode and it would be awful for you.

MS. N: You're right. I do have to watch *everything*. I watched him all the time. I think I always do that, to know whether the other person is going to hurt me.

THERAPIST: It must have been terrible to feel so helpless that you needed to do that! But now, when you watch things so very carefully, maybe the other person feels a bit as you did, when your father was checking up on every single thing you did.

MS. N: Huh. I never thought about it that way. But I don't think that this is anything that I can control. It's really too ingrained in me. And it's the only way I have to sort out what's going on with other people.

THERAPIST: Well, you did feel *so* hurt and frightened, it's understandable that you fear being hurt again. But that may be confusing or hurtful to *others*, that expectation. Our work is to sort this all out, so that you can discover when you *are* likely to be hurt and when your expectation of that is perhaps wrong, based on these experiences in the past with your father, rather than in the present with a different individual.

MS. N: I hope that will help. I don't like feeling that I'm pushing people away from me all the time, and maybe I am sometimes without knowing it. I just feel that people don't like me, and it makes me feel like a bad person.

The therapist's interpreting her patient's sense of fear and helplessness in these interactions first, before pointing out the reactive aggression in her dealings with others, helped Ms. N to feel understood and much less on the defensive. It also served to avoid an early enactment of the transference and countertransference feelings (Gabbard 1995). The therapist might have unthinkingly accepted the role of the judging, punishing parent by focusing on her patient's aggression in her dealings with others, without fully appreciating and interpreting the exquisite narcissistic vulnerability that was at its source. Ms. N would have only experienced such one-sided interpretations as another "beating," in which she was victimized and misunderstood yet again by an authority figure who did not fully realize how helpless and rejected she felt. This confirmation of her worst fears would have only served to escalate the patient's depression, rather than to help her more fully understand what was behind her self-destructive and provocative behavior.

Working With Dreams

Dreams provide a particular window into patients' unconscious fantasies and associative processes (Altman 1975; Blum 1976; Loden 2003). Working with dreams may help therapists gain information about their patients' defensive structure and unconscious wishes and fantasies and may help convince patients that ideas outside their awareness may exert a powerful effect on the way they think, perceive, and act.

For example, Dr. L, discussed earlier (see Case Example 4), had a recurrent dream in which a malevolent guided missile was soaring over the city where he worked and began to topple one of its most well-known buildings. (This dream occurred before September 11, 2001.) He was able to easily understand this dream on the basis of the work he was doing with his therapist about the kinds of humiliating attacks he expected chronically from the younger and older surgeons with whom he worked, as well as the kind of damage he feared he might do to others if he saw himself as a powerful man. Realizing that this dream connected to those fantasies provided him with even greater conviction about the pervasiveness of this unconscious fantasy.

Similarly, a 40-year-old opera singer, Ms. O, who experienced episodes of major depression, chronic dysthymia, and performance anxieties, benefited from dream work.

Case Example 7

Ms. O had a repeating dream that she dubbed the "I can't get there from here" dream. Usually it featured her being physically immobilized and unable to reach her dressing room or the stage. Ms. O readily identified the dream as connected with the inner sense of paralysis she experienced with her performance anxieties. Working with one particular variation on this dream, however, helped her to understand some of the conflicts behind these anxieties. In this version of the dream, a younger singer with whom she was actually competing for a part was featured. In this dream, Ms. O could not reach the stage because her path was blocked by the younger woman, who gestured to her belligerently. In another, related episode of the same dream, Ms. O herself was in prison for an unspecified crime.

Ms. O and her therapist had recently been discussing the patient's guilty memories of going to a dance shortly before her own mother died and of beginning to feel dismissively toward her mother about her lack of understanding of the patient's new relationships with boys. Ms. O had begun to realize that she always felt guilty and disloyal about living and having relationships and a successful career, whereas her mother, who had an unhappy and frustrated life, had died prematurely. In the context of these recent discoveries, and with the knowledge that the young woman in the dream was competing with Ms. O for a role, the therapist pointed out that the theme of guilt about outdoing her mother had found its way into the dream.

> THERAPIST: What stops you from "getting to where you need to be"—on the stage, performing—is your concern about aggression. The woman you are competing with in real life is aggressive toward you in the dream. But *you are the one to wind up in jail.* You get anxious about *your* aggression, about your desire to take the center stage and be seen there, alive and singing beautifully. So you stop yourself through your anxiety and your depression. You punish yourself for competing, which is too aggressive and disloyal! You think deep down that you should be in jail, not at the dance as your mother is dying, or performing now onstage.

Here, the context of the dream helps in understanding its particular meaning. The therapist considers the dynamic themes that are emerging during the treatment period in which the dream appears and also considers the day residue—that is, the daily events that appear in the dream and the thoughts the patient describes about them. In this dream, the day residue includes the fact that the woman in the dream is someone with whom Ms. O was competing that day for a job. It is helpful, in approaching a dream, to ask patients to talk about the different characters or activities in a dream and to mention any particular thoughts they may have about them. Obtaining these associations, along with thinking about the active themes in the treatment, helps to further illuminate the meanings of dreams. The therapist should not impose benchmark symbolic meanings. She rather uses the associations and context as the basis for interpretation.

Objectives of the Middle Phase of Treatment

By the time the middle phase is nearing an end, the extensive work with the patient's dynamics, described in more detail in the following chapters, results in a sense of comfort between patient and therapist that much has been understood about that patient's particular vulnerability to depressive affects. A reduction in the patient's sense of inadequacy or narcissistic vulnerability is noted, as is a reduction in reactive anger, in guilty self-recriminations, and in shameful self-appraisals. A diminished need to idealize others in order to feel better or to denigrate the self and others is also seen. This has been accomplished through dedicated work on the depressive dynamics as they occur in multiple settings, including in the transference.

The middle phase also offers the patient the repetitive experience of central core dynamic constellations. It makes familiar what was earlier unknown to consciousness and makes clear the restrictiveness and repetitiveness of these conflicts in the patient's life. In each of the following chapters, we illustrate therapeutic work in the middle phase, focusing on each of the central dynamics of depression and using the techniques described here.

References

Altman L: The Dream in Psychoanalysis. New York, International Universities Press, 1975

Blum H: The changing use of the dream in psychoanalytic practice. Int J Psychoanal 57:315–324, 1976 965166

Brenner C: Depressive affect, anxiety, and psychic conflict in the phallic-oedipal phase. Psychoanal Q 48(2):177–197, 1979 441209

Cooper AM: Changes in psychoanalytic ideas: transference interpretation. J Am Psychoanal Assoc 35(1):77–98, 1987 3584822

Gabbard GO: Sexual excitement and countertransference love in the analyst. J Am Psychoanal Assoc 42(4):1083–1106, 1994 7868782

Gabbard GO: Countertransference: the emerging common ground. Int J Psychoanal 76(Pt 3):475–485, 1995 7558607

Jacobs TJ: The inner experiences of the analyst: their contribution to the analytic process. Int J Psychoanal 74(Pt 1):7–14, 1993 8454406

Loden S: The fate of the dream in contemporary psychoanalysis. J Am Psychoanal Assoc 51(1):43–70, 2003 12731798

Makari G, Shapiro T: On psychoanalytic listening: language and unconscious communication. J Am Psychoanal Assoc 41(4):991–1020, 1993 8282944

Rothstein A, Chused J, Renik O, et al: Four aspects of the enactment concept: definitions, therapeutic effects, dangers, history. Journal of Clinical Psychoanalysis 8:9–79, 1999

Safran JD, Muran JC: Negotiating the Therapeutic Alliance. New York, Guilford, 2000

Sandler J: Countertransference and role-responsiveness. Int Rev Psychoanal 3:43–47, 1976

Searles HF: Oedipal love in the countertransference. Int J Psychoanal 40:180–190, 1959 14444362

Shapiro T: From monologue to dialogue: a transition in psychoanalytic practice. J Am Psychoanal Assoc 50(1):199–219, 2002 12018865

Stone L: Notes on the non-interpretive elements in the psychoanalytic situation and process (1981), in Transference and Its Context. New York, Jason Aronson, 1984, pp 153–176

Westen D, Gabbard GO: Developments in cognitive neuroscience: II. Implications for theories of transference. J Am Psychoanal Assoc 50(1):99–134, 2002 12018876

6

Addressing Narcissistic Vulnerability

NARCISSISTIC vulnerability is characterized by the tendency to react to slights and disappointments with a significant loss of self-esteem (Kohut 1966; Rothstein 1984; Spezzano 1993). As noted in Chapter 1 ("Introduction"), narcissistic vulnerability has been viewed by generations of analysts as central to the development of depression. Because of its crucial role, it is important to help the patient become aware of this vulnerability and to collaboratively explore its dynamics.

Narcissistic vulnerability is thought to arise in early experiences of helplessness, loss, or rejection, and temperamental factors may also play a role. The resulting sadness and feelings of being inadequate and unloved can be interpreted by these children as signs of personal damage or weakness. They may even experience their sadness and feelings of rejection somatically, as something physically wrong in the body, with the development of unconscious fantasies concerning bodily damage. If children envy others' strengths in contrast to the "damage" they imagine, this envy and associated anger may provide a further source of discomfort. They may feel even more unlovable, as they have aggressive feelings that seem toxic. Similarly, feelings of neediness linked to the experience of rejection may alarm children, who sense the burdens they place on the parent. The neediness is seen as something hard to manage or control, which will only distance needed caregivers. A sense of frustration and hopelessness becomes connected with the idea of actively seeking love and caring (Figure 6–1).

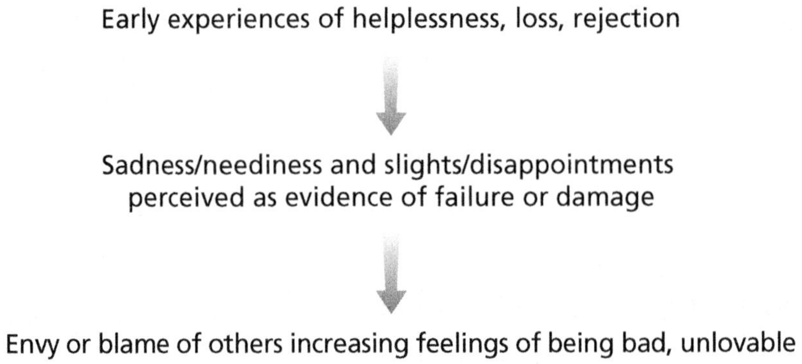

Early experiences of helplessness, loss, rejection

Sadness/neediness and slights/disappointments
perceived as evidence of failure or damage

Envy or blame of others increasing feelings of being bad, unlovable

Figure 6–1.   Narcissistic vulnerability.

If children experience these difficulties as immutable aspects of their identity from an early age, the early fantasies of failure and damage may persist or be easily evoked at later stages in life and dictate an affective response. When children enter the oedipal phase of development, for example, the expected competition with either parent for the other's love is stamped by the earlier patterned responses. Fantasies of love and longing that attach to the opposite-sex parent, with competition for his or her exclusive, romantically tinged love, is loosely called the *positive oedipal complex;* competition for the same-sex parent, the *negative oedipal complex.* If children, fearing that they are already damaged or too aggressive, retreat from these attempts at competition or experience this competition in a manner distorted by preexisting fears and doubts, there will be a lasting impact on their developing sense of masculine or feminine identity. Self-experience is contaminated with what Kilborne (2002) termed "oedipal shame," a conviction that the individual is deeply and essentially flawed, with accompanying fantasies of being too small, powerless, impotent, and weak. Such individuals feel too exposed to openly or successfully compete for love, admiration, or recognition (Kilborne 2002). Attempts to "disappear," to deny or to hide one's damage, result because relationships are interpreted as threatening sources of exposure. The self-experience of damage, exposure, or powerlessness can also distort the later development of a sense of autonomy, genuine relatedness, and independence in latency and adolescence, although this may always be subject to revision through strongly positive later experiences, including psychotherapy. It should be noted that these descriptions pertain to the "experienced" world of the child that is a composite of life events and subjective factors. This composite helps structure future experiences in semirigid templates that make life seem predictable but likely painful—these expectations are addressed by dynamic therapy.

For patients whose self-experience includes feeling damaged, helpless, or unlovable, slights and disappointments are internalized as confirmation of this shameful self-evaluation, triggering intense self-criticism and feelings of failure (Milrod 1988), in the form of a severe superego. These self-perceptions can rapidly generalize into a depressed mood state, as guilt about reactive anger (either envy of others, seen as more whole or more fortunate, or rage at those who have engendered helpless feelings) increases the depressive spiral through self-punishing actions (see depression cycle 1 [Figure 2–1] in Chapter 2, "Development of a Psychodynamic Model of Depression").

In this chapter, we illustrate how to explore and identify areas of narcissistic vulnerability common for depressed patients and offer case examples showing how to link these to perceptions of earlier life experiences. Then we discuss how to work with these realizations in treatment by 1) exploring the negative fantasies patients hold about themselves as a result of these areas of vulnerability, 2) connecting these fantasies to patients' sensitivity to rejection and disappointment to help them recognize their often distorted perceptions about others' response or about their own value, and 3) examining defensive responses to the vulnerabilities in patients' characteristic behavior that actually perpetuate intrapsychic conflict and frustration and disappointment in relationships.

Recognizing Areas of Narcissistic Vulnerability

In the following cases, the patients are helped to identify areas of narcissistic vulnerability and to understand the context in which such sensitivity or expectation of rejection may have developed. Common sources of such vulnerability include reactions to traumatic early separations, perceived rejection by a parent, a sense of helplessness and damage related to an early illness, and feelings of rejection because of perceived difference. Certain reactive fantasies that connect to these areas of vulnerability are also examined briefly.

Case Example 1: Understanding the Residues of Painful Childhood Separations

Ms. P presented with major depression and severe daily panic attacks during her final year in graduate school, when at age 30 she faced making decisions about where she would live in the future and about whether to continue a relationship with her boyfriend on whom she felt shamefully dependent. Her therapist noted that Ms. P tended to minimize any description of suffering or vulnerability and to feel deeply ashamed of her psychiatric illness, going to great lengths to hide it from anyone other than her therapist, parents, and boyfriend.

When this shame was explored, Ms. P associated to her feelings in childhood when she visited her father and stepmother. Ms. P was anxious when she was with them and apart from her mother and often had nightmares. Her stepmother had seemed unsympathetic, apparently viewing her anxiety states and nightmares as manipulative attempts to gain her father's attention, and her father seemed to go along with this perception. Ms. P viewed her anxiety states as deeply unacceptable.

Additionally, this young woman learned while in treatment that her mother had been depressed and preoccupied for a long time after her divorce from Ms. P's father, which had occurred when the patient was 6. Her mother admitted in retrospect that she had been emotionally rather unavailable to her daughter during the early years after the divorce. The patient had great difficulty remembering this; it seemed to remind her of a painful sadness that she retrospectively considered weak and terribly shameful.

In reaction to her feelings of sadness and longing for her mother's attention, it seemed that Ms. P had cultivated a compensatory sense of boyish invulnerability: She would not need anyone, as she had imagined was the case for some of the boisterous boys who were her playmates. Although she prided herself on being "like a guy," this adaptation made her feel rather deficient as a woman. Ms. P was very sensitive as an adolescent and young adult to her reception as a desirable woman by the young men she knew, and romantic rejections seemed to stir up all the sadness and painful longings that she had worked so hard to avoid. One of her problems with her current boyfriend was that she suspected she was staying with him only to avoid such painful rejections by other, more desirable men.

Exploration of this patient's sense of herself as defective because of understandable feelings of sadness and anxiety occurring in reaction to childhood experiences of emotional withdrawal, and identification of her reactive fantasies about herself as a boisterous boy versus an appealing woman, were decisive elements in helping her to recover from her depression.

Case Example 2: Identifying Feelings of Parental Rejection

Ms. Q, an artist in her 30s, was referred for treatment by her internist when she presented to him with a major depression after an abortive romantic relationship. Her lover, Jim, a married man, had been erratically attentive for a year, then abruptly terminated the relationship in a brusque but joking manner that she found especially painful. When asked to think about her reaction to this particular behavior, she immediately identified the sense of pain as connected to her relationship with her father. A gambler and philanderer, her father would often leave the family for brief periods, only to reappear with a joking demeanor that made light of his wife's and children's upset about his abandonment of them. His joking and teasing were impossible to penetrate and thus maddening. Nonetheless, they seemed preferable to Ms. Q to her mother's bitter sense of victimization, and Ms. Q struggled constantly for his approval with her own flippant, upbeat style. However, "it always felt like maybe I could fight to capture his attention for two minutes, and that would be it."

Ms. Q's mother seemed consistently overwhelmed by the demands of raising her five children and offered little recognition of her daughter, either. The high-spirited patient managed to find ways of entertaining her siblings and friends, somewhat as her father, when present, entertained the family, and this became a significant source of self-esteem. In adulthood, however, after a number of love relationships failed, Ms. Q found that this technique was wearing thin. It had not managed to keep Jim connected to her, despite his frequent comments about how similar they were to one another, with their wit and verve, paired with a significant vulnerability. Ms. Q began to feel contempt for these aspects of herself (identified with her father) but also hated herself for her increasing depression, feeling that it made her "a completely unlovable victim," like her mother.

Ms. Q, a quite insightful woman, had been already aware of the similarities between Jim and her father. However, she was helped a good deal in her treatment when she began to recognize that her painful feelings of rejection by both parents had resulted in the internalization of a sense that she was "either too much" (that her needs of others were overwhelming) or "too little" (that she was inadequate as a woman) for anyone to genuinely love her. Her ability to realize that this powerful, internalized fantasy was untrue, by way of her relationship with her therapist and especially through interpretations of the transference, was essential in her recovery from depression. Thus recovery was dependent on easing her rigid perceptive set.

Case Example 3: Identifying Vulnerability Based on Perceived Difference

Mr. R was a highly successful architect in his 40s when he presented for treatment for depression, which had been apparently triggered by a crisis in his relationship with his same-sex partner, Sam. The pair had been together for 3 years, but Sam described an increasing dissatisfaction with their sexual relationship, in which Mr. R was quite inhibited.

In discussing the relationship, Mr. R's feelings about his desirability and about his own sexual desires were explored. Mr. R reported a sense of shame and distress about his homosexuality, of which he had been at least partially aware from early childhood. Mr. R also described being teased from early on by his father and two brothers for his differences in temperament and behavior.

> MR. R: I would go and decorate my room when I was upset—you know, I would rearrange the furniture—sort of my way of keeping control. This seemed just incomprehensible to them, a big joke. It was really very hurtful. Like there was something about me that they just couldn't ever accept. I was a large child, and I couldn't be physically bullied, but I was teased—a lot—by the three of them, and it always felt terrible.

This teasing, which Mr. R gradually identified as directed at his different kind of masculinity, combined with the strict religious prohibitions on most forms of sexuality that characterized his upbringing, led this patient to feel deeply rejected, hurt, and defensive about his sexuality. The current situation with his partner provided an opportunity to address a sense of hopelessness about ever being accepted sexually or accepting his sexuality himself.

Case Example 4: Identifying the Legacy of a Life-Threatening Childhood Illness

Ms. S was an energetic young college student of 20, inclined to be moody, who characteristically dealt with her fears and conscious sense of shyness by pushing herself to encounter physical challenges in sports and to engage socially with others. She was seen as athletic and "tough" by her peers. In her junior year, Ms. S experienced an acute bout of appendicitis, which resulted in surgery. During her hospitalization, she began to experience an overwhelming sense of depression, which led her doctors to request psychiatric consultation for her.

During the consultation, Ms. S was asked how she viewed her current, relative physical helplessness. She immediately burst into tears. "All my life, I have avoided feeling helpless. I just can't accept this, even though I know that that is crazy and that this is only temporary. It has always felt completely necessary to me to feel that I can do anything, physically speaking."

Ms. S noted that since the surgery, she had begun having powerful memories of being held down to have medical treatments when she was a child. When she asked her parents about this, they described her chemotherapy and radiation treatments for a childhood cancer when she was 3 years old. Her parents had never withheld this information from Ms. S; she had been aware of her childhood cancer diagnosis but had fiercely avoided discussing it with them until the present.

A series of therapeutic interviews, followed by psychotherapy, helped Ms. S to understand that her sense of having been acutely helpless and desperately ill during this prolonged childhood experience had remained with her in persistent, unconscious fantasies of shameful damage and life-threatening vulnerability that she kept trying relentlessly to disprove to herself and others. Recognizing the pervasiveness and power of these fantasies eventually helped Ms. S to understand her driven and perfectionistic athleticism. Her moodiness was understood as a response to any hint of vulnerability on her part, and her depression—a significant one, which had persisted for several weeks and been accompanied by a suicidal gesture—was understood as an overwhelming response to the sense of helplessness and rage evoked by the current illness and its treatment.

Understanding Distortions in Self-Image and in Perceptions of Others

We now explore how to work with these initial recognitions to help patients become aware of the ways in which such vulnerabilities lead them to distort their experiences of themselves and of others (Table 6–1). These interpretations are based on internalized models of self and others as described by Bowlby and others (see Chapter 2). Understanding these distortions opens a pathway for later exploration of the varied adaptations these patients have made in their lives, often on the basis of such distortions, which they find deeply frustrating and often shameful.

Ms. H, the lawyer described in Chapter 4 ("Getting Started With Psychodynamic Treatment of Depression"; see Case Example 5) as having become depressed after her breakup, at age 38, with her boyfriend of 5 years, represents a good example of a patient who at times misinterpreted herself and others from the standpoint of how "pathetic and humiliated" she seemed in comparison to others, judged as "cool."

Case Example 5A

An example of Ms. H's misinterpretations of herself and others occurred after her former boyfriend contacted her, admitting that he was in pain about

Table 6–1.   Treating narcissistic vulnerability

1. Identify sources—experiences of illness, separation, rejection, difference—
    and related fantasies about the self.

2. Help patient recognize distortions in perception of self and others.

3. Recognize reactive, counterproductive fantasies, defenses, and behaviors.

their parting and about the callous way in which he had initiated it. Ms. H
waited to collect her thoughts, then commented on what she had begun to
learn in her treatment were problematic aspects of the relationship, apart
from the issue of disagreeing about marriage and children. After discussing
this in a fairly controlled manner, she responded to his wishes to "try again"
by an indication that she might consider this, if he agreed to enter a conjoint
therapy in which they could be helped to face their difficulties.

Once he had established that Ms. H might be willing to try again, however, her boyfriend balked and retreated, saying that perhaps he "needed to
do some work" on his own before he could think about returning and that
he would think about it and "maybe be in touch." Ms. H was, by turns, flab-
bergasted, furious, and then devastated about this turn of events. By the
time she came to her treatment session, she was sobbing, disconsolate, and
self-critical.

> MS. H: The worst part of it was, I completely humiliated myself.
>   I should have known better. It must have looked as if I were
>   pleading with him. He hates that. It makes me seem incred-
>   ibly unattractive.
> THERAPIST: How do you figure that?
> MS. H: He always talked about how he hated being the one with
>   all the power in the relationship.
> THERAPIST: Can you tell me how you saw him as powerful in this
>   conversation?
> MS. H: Well, I know he is a jerk. But he comes off being the one
>   to reject me, always, even after it seemed that he wanted to
>   get back together.
> THERAPIST: And you think he rejected you because he was feeling
>   powerful and seeing you as weak?
> MS. H: Yes. It's always been like that with him. It's so frustrating, it's
>   unbelievable. I wish I had just left it that I'd think about it,
>   and tormented *him* for a change. I'm too honest. It's really pa-
>   thetic. That's what I mean about other women being able to
>   seem more…mysterious. It works for them. I just can't do it.

The therapist decided here to actively pursue Ms. H's fantasy that her
boyfriend was very powerful, especially because it connected to her perva-

sive sense of continually being humiliated, as well as not so mysterious (read: powerful and captivating) as other women.

> THERAPIST: It sounded to me as if you were simply doing what it takes to engage in a relationship! I'm not sure, from what you describe, that Tom knows how to do that. That doesn't seem especially powerful to me. I am intrigued by your thought that you seemed pathetic. What's pathetic about what you did or said?
>
> MS. H: It's just that...I wind up feeling sad and miserable, and Tom just...looks cool. I'll never find a man, feeling so sad and hurt, and he will just go ahead and find someone else, since he thinks he's perfectly fine.
>
> THERAPIST: It sounds as if maybe Tom and you share the fantasy that it's pathetic to really care or to need someone. It makes both of you very frightened and uncomfortable. He tries to shrug off that feeling, or to transfer it to you, and you feel...as if you are left holding the bag...and that makes you pathetic. Do you really believe that? Have you felt this way in other relationships?

Here the therapist used a mentalizing approach to explore what might be motivating Tom that was different from Ms. H's rigid expectations. Questioning Ms. H about other relationships represented a further attempt to educate her about her pattern of current misperceptions. It also might have helped Ms. H to link current distortions to the childhood experiences that mobilized persistent, unconscious fantasies about herself in adulthood.

> MS. H [*after a long pause*]: I think I felt this sometimes with my brothers. They were older and seemed...so cool. They could do so many things I couldn't. I wanted to be with them, and if I acted a certain way—you know, always doing what they wanted, making them feel good, being funny and wild—it worked out. But when I couldn't be that way, it just...didn't. The worst thing I could do was to look like I *needed* them to play with me. That made them—and it certainly made me—feel that I was a complete loser.

The therapist then pointed to the unrealistic aspects of this interpretation of events and linked it, by use of genetic interpretation, to other historical material that they had discussed and that also contributed to this patient's vulnerability.

> THERAPIST: In fact, your brothers were a lot older than you. It's no wonder that you couldn't always keep up or that they didn't

always want to play with you! And your mother sounds as if she were preoccupied with her own concerns, and your father, off in his own world. But it was probably hard for you to realize that there were reasons that you weren't really…seen or recognized for yourself…that had very little to do with you. To avoid maybe feeling sad or upset about all that, you would do anything to connect. You could be really entertaining! But deep down, that didn't always make you feel good, either.

MS. H: I guess that's probably true. When I would try so hard to connect to them, it felt like I couldn't really be me. I think the humiliating part was that I felt, to be accepted, that I would have to make myself into something else for them. I do that so much, and whenever I do it, I hate myself. But I have also always hated myself when I feel sad. That's probably even worse for me. It just feels so awful.

THERAPIST: It seems as if you are doing the same thing now. Instead of just seeing Tom as a man with a lot of difficulty loving someone and yourself as a woman who was trying to be involved in a caring relationship, you think of yourself as a loser and him as cool, together, and rejecting—the way you see your brothers. And you feel like a sad person whom no one will ever want, as if that were a fact of your existence, or your destiny, rather than realizing that you've had those feelings for real reasons.

MS. H: I just hate feeling that I can't control things!

Her therapist underscored reality versus fantasy one last time, in an empathic fashion:

THERAPIST: It's really, really hard when things aren't in your control. But you wind up interpreting that as connected to something missing *in* you, or wrong *with* you, rather than seeing and accepting this as something outside of yourself.

The insights developed in this session needed to be worked through exhaustively in this treatment. It became apparent from this interchange as well as from other, later discussions, that Ms. H's feeling that she could never completely hold the attention of her parents or of her brothers was ensconced in her fantasies of being deficient. For this patient, these fantasies connected particularly to her sexuality. Ms. H felt both deficiently feminine—not mysterious or powerful, as she saw some women—*and* deficiently masculine, as contrasted to her boisterous and competent older brothers, to whom her mother was very drawn. The fact that Ms. H did not see her mother as powerfully feminine, either, but thought her incapable of capturing her elusive father's interest, seemed to contribute further to fantasies of deficiency. Ms. H felt identified with her mother and was likely frightened of competing with her for feminine "power," because her mother was the one parent who was rather consistently available. This was another potential dynamic: the need to see herself as inadequate to avoid her competitiveness damaging her mother.

When Ms. H chose an emotionally rather unavailable man to love, she seemed to be partly motivated by oedipal factors—choosing a familiar love object, someone quite different in personality from her father but actually very much like him in his emotional distance. Further, Ms. H perceived herself to be a sad, yearning, and deficient being who needed to gain power through her connection with a "cool," powerful man, Tom, who seemed on the face of things to have no such needs. Losing this man meant that she was consigned to be, again, a sad, deficient, humiliated "loser." This left Ms. H feeling hopeless and depressed. This represents another dynamic found in these patients, corresponding to depression cycle 2 (Figure 2–2) from Chapter 2. Ms. H's attempt to be involved with a man whom she idealized represented an effort to compensate for feelings of inadequacy. However, this led to an unrealistic perception of him with recurrent disappointments and self-devaluation for not being able to maintain his interest.

Much of the work of this treatment involved a multilayered exploration of these fantasies, related to Ms. H's central areas of narcissistic vulnerability. Work would obviously be done, too, with her rage at the frustrating people whom she loved and about her associated guilt for this anger. Dealing with angry reactions to narcissistic injury is explored in detail in Chapter 7 ("Addressing Angry Reactions to Narcissistic Injury"). Here, we present therapeutic work that helped Ms. H consider how her defensive responses to this sense of vulnerability sometimes worked against the establishment of the secure relationships that she craved.

Understanding Counterproductive Reactions to Narcissistic Vulnerability

Persistent early fantasies and the feelings that become connected to them are often characteristically resisted or expressed in ways that become embedded in a patient's repertoire of responses to relationships and to attempts at self-expression. For example, Arieti and Bemporad (1978) wrote of a tendency they found in their depressed patients to continually attempt to gain security from parents who had unrealistically high expectations of them. To avoid the sadness and sense of inadequacy their parents' unrealistic expectations engendered, these patients would characteristically come to conform to their parents' wishes and try to please them, even by substantially inhibiting their own desires. The need to do this in order to maintain a close connection to the parents, and the need to bury guilt-inducing, frightening reactive anger, became a way of life. In adulthood, these depressed patients would continue to search for connection with "dominant others," from whom they would again seek approval and recognition. When these others became disaffected or rejected the patient, however, it felt intolerable and would trigger depression. In another vein, Brenner (1975) wrote of patients whose lifelong attempts to minimize the sadness, shame, and painful affects connected to their sense that they were inferior led them to inhibit and constrict their desires. In either case, lifelong adaptations develop that are ultimately quite frustrating for patients and only further their sense of basic inadequacy. It is important to explore these frustrating and embedded character patterns with patients, both in terms of their history and their current relationships and in the transference.

Ms. H, whose case was discussed earlier (see Case Example 5A), became involved in an exploratory process with her therapist when she recognized that she seemed, in many of her relationships, to be craving connection and working overtime with fairly frustrating people to gain it. This continued to be a theme in much of her therapeutic work. As noted earlier, one aspect of this connected to Ms. H's fantasies of being deficient and seeking connections with "powerful" men and women through which she would no longer feel so helpless, the dynamic of compensatory idealization described above. Another salient aspect of Ms. H's difficulties in relationships concerned her desperate effort not to feel sad or alone, because these feelings suggested to her that she was damaged. She interpreted those feelings as evidence of humiliation and powerlessness and had a frantic need to avoid them. Additionally, Ms. H had difficulty being directly and effectively angry with those whom she loved, feeling safer articulating anger about others to whom she was not so attached. Because of this difficulty and because she was averse to presenting herself as hurt or sad, Ms. H sometimes portrayed herself as the righteously angry (though not sad or hurt) victim of others.

Case Example 5B

Ms. H was struggling with her disappointment about the actions of a partner in her legal firm and with her relationship with Susan, a friend at her firm whom Ms. H had initially idealized.

Ms. H: I'm disappointed in Susan. She is turning out to be such a flake. I tried to talk with her about my problems with the partner I'm working for yesterday, but she turned it around and blamed me.

THERAPIST: Can you tell me more about that?

Ms. H: He picked an associate with less experience for a case, and I was complaining about it to her. A lot of other people mentioned that they were upset for me, and I got really angry. I think she knows that I'm right, but she looks up to this partner and doesn't want to hear anything bad about him. So she basically told me to drop it.

THERAPIST: You've mentioned something like this with her before. Do you think it makes her upset when you get so angry at him?

Ms. H: I guess so.

THERAPIST: It sounded before like she gets anxious when you're angry about things, and that she does always tend to defend your boss. That may be an issue of hers. But before you got so angry, my sense is that you actually felt hurt and overlooked when the other associate was chosen to do the work. Do you know why it's hard for you to talk with Susan about *those* feelings?

Ms. H: I hate feeling like that! It makes me seem like such a loser.

THERAPIST: We've talked before about how much you hate feeling sad, because it makes you feel so vulnerable. You can't imagine that other people will be drawn to you when you feel that way. But I think that when you limit your range of feeling so much, it has the opposite effect. You seem unforgiving when in fact you are simply reacting to how hurt and sad you are. About Susan: you *do* seem to automatically interpret what your boss did as a humiliation, rather than a decision you don't understand and have to work out with him. Do you think that she might be reacting to that as well?

Ms. H: I don't know about that. I think she is just sucking up to the partner, which is something that really bothers me about her. But I do think you have a point. I need to talk with him about what he decided. And I know that I feel really humiliated about everything. I guess that does happen a lot with me.

In this vignette, we see that Ms. H avoided expressing hurt feelings that evoked for her a sense of damage or humiliation. The therapist gently confronted the patient with her tendency to avoid direct and potentially clarifying expressions of anger toward those with whom she was in conflict, her avoidance of revealing hurt and disappointment, and her reaction to disappointment instead with feelings of victimization. The way in which she attempted to enlist her peers in this sense of victimization sometimes distanced others.

Ms. G, whose case was described in Chapter 4 (see Case Examples 4A and 4B in that chapter) as the journalist who was depressed during a time when her boyfriend felt distant and uninvolved, had also developed maladaptive behavior patterns.

Case Example 6

Ms. G's mother had been ill during her teenage years, and this patient had felt alone. She was angry about her father's reliance on her to take care of the house and about his failure to recognize her feelings of loss and anxiety during her mother's illness and her need to continue her studies at that time. These events reinforced an earlier feeling that her father favored his male students (her father was a college professor and had developed close relationships with a number of his male students, often inviting them to dinner), while overlooking her own talents and abilities. Her sense of deep injury led Ms. G to expect that others, especially men, would similarly overlook her achievements.

At work, this patient developed a style of rigid insistence on being recognized for her position of authority, alternating with self-punishing retreats into feelings of paralysis when she was especially angry about her appraisal by the predominantly male hierarchy in her department. In her relationship, Ms. G felt helpless and frequently hurt by her boyfriend's distance and interpreted it almost exclusively as a humiliating rejection. This led her to icily distance herself, in turn, from him.

> MS. G [*tearfully*]: I don't know why I am so upset. But I feel like work is a nightmare. No one there will ever see what I can do, because they don't respect me. I see that and get tongue-tied. It becomes a self-fulfilling prophecy.
>
> THERAPIST: You do seem convinced that no one will ever see how competent you are. And we've seen how much this echoes your feelings about your father. When you talk about a self-fulfilling prophecy, I wonder. Are you so sure, really, that you are seen as badly as you imagine?
>
> MS. G: I don't know. I do realize that I am used to seeing myself as powerless, and I know, from the things we've talked about, that that isn't always the case. It's hard to imagine that I have an impact on anyone.
>
> THERAPIST: Can you give me an example of something that upset you recently at work?
>
> MS. G: Well, Adam just went over my head the other day the other day and spoke with my boss instead of me. He didn't even

consult me about a fairly important matter, and he should have. What does he think of me, that he doesn't talk with me first?

THERAPIST: You and he have had some problems lately, I know. But I wonder if that might be part of it. You are convinced that he overlooks you out of disdain and contempt. But maybe he doesn't feel so comfortable with you, and turns to your boss for help instead, because he feels less exposed in front of him. Maybe he is not so much disdainful as anxious.

MS. G: I know that you were saying that about Michael [her boyfriend] the other day. And I did think that you might be right. I am so hurt by him that I just hold back, and I never even think that that might have an impact on *him*. But the other day, I snapped at him, and his eyes welled up with tears. It's so hard for me to imagine that *my* withdrawal or *my* anger has an impact on him, but they clearly do!

Here, the therapist pointed to Ms. G's distortions of others' actions based on her tendency to feel humiliated with men, linked this to her historical sense of injury in the relationship with her father, and examined how her reactive withdrawal and iciness could alienate the men in her life now. Ms. G's characteristic attempts to avoid her painful and angry feelings led her to project the anger and self-condemnation onto others. By doing that, she felt less aggressive, but ashamed and vulnerable as she experienced herself as rejected by others. This combination of guilt over her aggression and her susceptibility to shame led to a self-punishing "paralysis." All of that, taken together, created the "self-fulfilling prophecy" of which patient and therapist spoke. Because these issues had been examined many times together in the treatment, the therapist was able to fairly quickly address these issues with this patient. At this point, in the early middle phase of her treatment, Ms. G still had great difficulty in speaking about her feelings about her therapist, and transference interpretations did not become a prominent part of the treatment until later in the therapy. At that point, her shame about her dependent feelings toward the therapist, and her fear that these would seem disgusting or childish and provoke abandonment, were actively addressed.

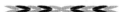

In summary, identifying the developmental origins of the sense of vulnerability, recognizing the fantasies that connect to it, and identifying the reactive envy or blame to which this gives rise is an important task of the beginning and middle phases of the treatment. Helping patients to recognize distortions in perception that stem from narcissistic vulnerability, both in their life and in the transference relationship, and to also recognize counterproductive behaviors and defenses related to it, are essential components of any psychodynamic treatment of depression.

References

Arieti S, Bemporad J: Severe and Mild Depression: The Psychotherapeutic Approach. New York, Basic Books, 1978

Brenner C: Affects and psychic conflict. Psychoanal Q 44(1):5–28, 1975 1114198

Kilborne B: Disappearing Persons: Shame and Appearance. Albany, State University of New York Press, 2002

Kohut H: Forms and transformations of narcissism. J Am Psychoanal Assoc 14(2): 243–272, 1966 5941052

Milrod D: A current view of the psychoanalytic theory of depression. With notes on the role of identification, orality, and anxiety. Psychoanal Study Child 43:83–99, 1988 3067251

Rothstein A: The Narcissistic Pursuit of the Transference, 2nd Edition, Revised. New York, International Universities Press, 1984

Spezzano C: Affect in Psychoanalysis: A Clinical Synthesis. Hillsdale, NJ, Analytic Press, 1993

Addressing Angry Reactions to Narcissistic Injury

TYPICALLY, patients respond to narcissistic injury with angry reactions and fantasies (Jacobson 1971; Rado 1928; Stone 1986). They tend to have difficulty tolerating these aggressive feelings and may deny them. In attempting to approach the reactive anger, it is essential that the therapist take a nonjudgmental stance, because patients are often critical of these feelings and expect a negative reaction from others.

It is important in treating depression psychodynamically to explore angry reactions to perceived rejections in early life, as well as negative affects toward those with whom the patient has experienced a recent loss or rejection (Abraham 1911, 1924; see Chapter 2, "Development of a Psychodynamic Model of Depression"). Jealousy and vengefulness may also emerge in the context of narcissistic injury, because patients will covet what others have and what they feel deprived of. Therapeutic efforts are aimed at helping patients become more tolerant of and less threatened by their anger and jealousy, which they tend to see as disruptive to relationships and potentially harmful to others (Table 7–1). In addition, angry and vengeful feelings and fantasies can trigger guilt and may cause a lowering of self-esteem. Anger often is turned toward the self, intensifying depressive symptoms. As patients explore origins of their rageful, jealous, or spiteful affects and realize the distortions in perception these often cause, these feelings become "detoxified." They are no longer dreaded or disowned as unacceptable reactions that will ensure rejection or condemnation.

Table 7–1.   Working with angry reactions to narcissistic injury

Areas of exploration

1. Addressing a lack of awareness of anger
2. Identifying specific angry fantasies
3. Identifying guilty reactions to anger
4. Identifying expectations of punishment
5. Exploring the link between competitiveness and aggression
6. Becoming more comfortable with assertiveness
7. Recognizing anger directed toward the self

Anticipated response to exploration

1. Increased comfort with assertiveness
2. Diminished self-directed anger

Addressing a Lack of Awareness of Anger

Sometimes patients with depression are unaware of experiencing any anger toward others. As noted previously, they may avoid the knowledge or experience of anger through a variety of defense mechanisms, including denial and repression, projection of angry feelings externally, reaction formation, or passive aggression, which can then exacerbate depression. Depressive symptoms in and of themselves can lead to avoidance of the experience of anger, as feelings of hopelessness or sadness predominate. Additionally, because of their low self-esteem and conflicts, depressed patients may feel they "don't have a right" to be angry. The appearance or expression of helplessness and passivity can allow depressed patients to deny hostility and aggressive intent.

Case Example 1A

Mr. T was a 62-year-old salesman who presented with a major depression of moderate intensity, connected to his fears about aging. He was experiencing uncharacteristic difficulties with his job, having lost several of his accounts, and began to fear that his age was a factor in this decline. Many of Mr. T's previous sales contacts had retired or moved to other locations, and he was no longer afforded the respect or responsiveness he had received in the past. In addition, he worried that his wife, who was 20 years younger, might no longer be sexually interested in him. She seemed much less passionate in their lovemaking and wanted to have sex less often than usual.

In addition, Mr. T experienced problems with his potency, which he also attributed to aging, and feared that this was driving his wife away. He suspected her of having an affair but was wary about bringing it up. He noticed that she was often away from the house engaging in somewhat mysterious activities, especially when he was traveling for business. Nevertheless, she seemed to enjoy being with him and expressed frustration with his frequent need to travel. He reported that he was not particularly angry with her, because he understood why she would be less interested in an aging man like him. He felt he should not confront her, partly because of this "understanding" and partly because he deeply feared the hurt of learning that she was involved with someone else.

The therapist felt that Mr. T was in denial about his anger at his wife and that he demonstrated a degree of reaction formation in his ready acceptance of her hurtful behavior. The therapist began to tentatively approach this with the patient.

> THERAPIST: It seems surprising, given your wife's behavior, that you would not feel more anger toward her.
>
> MR. T: Well, I'm not sure I have a right to be angry. I don't know that I can expect more. I'm not the man I used to be. As I told you, sometimes I can't even get an erection.
>
> THERAPIST: Have you been angry at her about other issues?
>
> MR. T: Well, about 10 years ago, I did find out she was having an affair. I was furious with her and threatened divorce. She became very upset about this possibility and really changed her behavior. She became warmer again, and things seem to be go very well again until about a year ago.
>
> THERAPIST: Then it seems even more surprising, since you were so angry about similar behavior in the past.
>
> MR. T: As I say, things were different then. I was younger. I was very successful at work.

Mr. T's diminished standing at work was particularly troubling to him. His loss of accounts led to threats of being fired from his job. Although he had enough money to retire, he feared a loss of purpose in not having his work. He described how his parents were always critical of his capabilities when he was young and said that he saw his earlier work successes as a way of demonstrating that they were wrong. He experienced long-standing feelings of inadequacy and unmanliness, for which work had partially compensated.

The therapist suggested to him that his old feelings of inadequacy were returning in the setting of his current difficulties performing at work.

Mr. T then presented a dream in which he saw a masseuse on a train who handed him a key. In the next scene, he was sitting with the masseuse and his wife at a table. Another man came up to his wife and hit her. The therapist suspected that the dream indicated something about the patient's dis-

connection from his anger at his wife—that Mr. T was the "other man" who
hit his wife. In associating to the dream, the patient revealed that he had occasionally been going to masseuses for sexual satisfaction.

> THERAPIST: I think this is another indication that you are angrier
>   at your wife than you thought.
> MR. T: Yes. I think I've been becoming more aware of that lately.
>   I'm upset that I've put up with these limitations on our sexual
>   activity! Sometimes she's willing to have sex only once every
>   couple of weeks.

The therapist considered that the dream may also have transference implications. Is the therapist the masseuse giving him the key to unlock access
to his feelings? Giving him the key to restore his potency? Although he
thought it was premature to suggest a transference interpretation, the therapist kept it in mind as a potential theme in the relationship.

Mr. T denied feeling anger at his mother as well, despite both his parents'
apparent favoring of his older brother. His parents praised his brother's
strength and athleticism, while having little that was positive to say about the
patient. His father paid much greater attention to the brother, both positive
and negative. When in conflict, the father and brother would get into near
violent fights. Mr. T felt that his mother was his only support in the troubled
family, even though this support was limited. In fact, Mr. T felt he could re-
tain her love only if he submitted to her insistent pressure on him to be the
"good" son. In contrast, both parents seemed preoccupied with, and perhaps
vicariously stimulated by, his brother's unruliness. In essence, Mr. T felt that
castration—essentially a diminution in his sense of masculinity and autonomy—was required for his mother's attention and approval.

On further questioning, Mr. T revealed more anger at his mother than
he had initially been able to indicate. He felt his mother had pressured him
to marry his first wife, about whom he had been very ambivalent, and with
whom he had been increasingly unhappy. In addition, the mother had never
adequately addressed the seriousness of his brother's problems, which included alcoholism and difficulty maintaining a job.

Mr. T's increasing awareness of his anger, then, allowed him to comprehend the need to more directly address certain problems with his wife. As
is described below in continuations of this case history, his wife was actually
quite responsive to these confrontations, easing his depression.

Identifying Specific Angry Fantasies

As noted in the opening of this chapter, the anger of depressed patients is
typically a response to their feelings of narcissistic injury. These angry reac-

tions can include bitterness about feeling unloved, vengeful feelings toward parents or siblings who were abusive, jealousy of those who are better off, and envying others their success, happier families, better health, better looks, or confidence.

Despite the specificity of their angry reactions, depressed patients are often vague about the content of their aggressive feelings and fantasies. Angry fantasies are typically unique and meaningful for each patient. Therefore, it is of value for the therapist to elicit their specific content. Because patients are often guilty about, ashamed of, or fearful of their angry fantasies, they may be reluctant to be forthcoming. Nevertheless, with ongoing exploration, and in the context of a therapeutic alliance and an increasing sense of safety with the therapist, patients usually reveal the specific contents of their feelings.

Case Example 2

Ms. U, a 49-year-old computer technician struggling with depressive symptoms, described an incident in which she had become angry with her close friend, Jennifer. She admitted to Jennifer that she was very upset about turning 50, particularly because she was unmarried and childless; she felt like a failure. Jennifer, who was somewhat older, responded that she should quit wallowing in her misery and "get over it." Ms. U was furious, particularly as she recalled helping her friend through a "midlife crisis" when Jennifer had turned 50 a few years before. However, Ms. U did not reveal her feelings to her friend. That night, the patient reported that she had a dream in which her younger sister committed suicide.

In associating to the dream, Ms. U described the history of her sister's difficulties. Her sister had a poorly identified mental illness, possibly schizophrenia, and her condition had deteriorated steadily over time. She was unemployed and had almost no friends. Ms. U recalled being both embarrassed by her sister during her childhood and jealous and angry about the attention that she received because of her problems. The patient felt that her parents, preoccupied with her sister's troubles, had little time for her and little interest.

Her therapist felt it might be useful to explore her dream to get further information about her fantasies. Ms. U's therapeutic work had already helped her identify and tolerate feelings of rage, but she also continued to struggle with them.

> THERAPIST: What comes to mind about the dream?
> Ms. U: I was scared at times that my sister might commit suicide, but I also think I wanted to be rid of her. It's upsetting to consider, but maybe I had wishes to kill her off. And maybe I wanted to kill Jennifer.

THERAPIST: I think that makes sense. It seems as if you were mur-
derously angry! I wonder if being so angry now at Jennifer,
for her lack of attention to your problems, reminds you of
how angry you always felt toward your sister, since your parents paid so much attention to her and not to you.

MS. U: That's true. Because of all the attention she got, I was always
jealous and angry with my sister. I was mean to her! Then, I
would worry that I had something to do with her problems.

THERAPIST: It seems like you felt really ignored emotionally by
Jennifer, just as you felt with your family.

MS. U: It did feel like that. But wanting to get rid of my sister or
Jennifer makes me feel guilty.

THERAPIST: I guess these wishes show just how hurt and angry you
felt growing up.

The emergence of these specific fantasies helped her therapist to understand more about Ms. U's sense of narcissistic injury. This patient had felt
neglected by her parents, because they focused so much attention on her sister, and embarrassed by her sibling's unusual behavior. The therapist's understanding helped the patient to gradually accept the anger and guilt that had
flourished in her family environment. Further, the therapist's nonjudgmental
stance helped Ms. U to reveal her childhood wishes that her sister might successfully commit suicide or to murder her sister and to begin to experience
these vengeful wishes as comprehensible and hence as less guilt-provoking
and toxic.

Identifying Guilty Reactions to Anger

Aggression and associated affects and fantasies can trigger intense guilt, making it sometimes intolerable for patients to discuss or admit to their anger,
especially because they may view this feeling as hurtful or damaging to
those they love. Sometimes the guilt is so pervasive that patients may not
immediately acknowledge it. Handling the guilt stimulated by aggressive
reactions to narcissistic injury is discussed at greater length in Chapter 8
("The Severe Superego and Guilt"). Here, case examples are offered that illustrate the value of identifying patients' angry reactions that stimulate guilt.
Helping patients to acknowledge the difference between angry thoughts and
fantasies and actual aggressive actions is of great importance here, in that the
guilt associated with such thoughts is often as intense for depressed patients
as if they had actually committed the imagined actions.

Case Example 1B

Mr. T described how he felt jealous about his parents favoring his older brother, who was bigger, tougher, and more gregarious than the patient. This brother would become involved in frequent scrapes with the law and often hit or insulted Mr. T. As a boy, the patient felt enraged but did not confront his sibling, because of a fear of his prowess and a reluctance to disappoint their mother's view of him as the "good son." Over time, however, his brother became an alcoholic and struggled professionally. His tendency to fight and argue with bosses had led to a series of job losses, and he was in financially tenuous circumstances. Mr. T felt guilty that somehow he had contributed to his brother's problems.

Mr. T saw his brother as failing in his life, and in treatment he was helped to understand the frightening, guilty pleasure that he experienced about this failure and to realize that his feelings did not mean that he had actually caused his brother's difficulties.

Case Example 3

Ms. V, a 25-year-old who was working at an advertising agency, had been exploring feelings of rejection by her father that were an important source of her depression. The father had left home when she was 4 years old and had little contact with the family. Her mother had been very disparaging of him and complained frequently about his abandonment of the family. Ms. V had little recollection of anger at her father and mainly recalled intense longings for his approval and wishes he would visit her. However, she had recently been increasingly aware of her anger at him as she explored the issue further in her therapy. In particular, she had been recalling the intensity of pain she had experienced at her father's lack of effort to maintain any consistent contact with her. In addition, her father was highly secretive about his life. The patient often did not know where he was, and at one point he revealed, several months after the event, that he had married.

> MS. V: I realize that I am actually very angry at my father, but it's very difficult to talk about it.
> THERAPIST: What makes it so hard?
> MS. V: It feels way too harsh.
> THERAPIST: Do you think you feel guilty or embarrassed about having these feelings toward him?
> MS. V: Yes, I do. I mean my mother was right about his abandoning us, but she was always so angry at him. I loved him and wanted to be with him. Maybe he was doing the best that he could do. He went through a lot when he was growing up.

THERAPIST: Well, he certainly may have been affected by his background, but I think it's still important to understand your
feelings toward him. Also, you may be emphasizing his background because you feel guilty about how angry you are.

MS. V: I also think you'll see me as an unforgiving and harsh person.

THERAPIST: It seems as if you expect me to feel critical of your feelings just as you do.

MS. V: It's hard to admit that sometimes these feelings are really
strong. I think that what I really want is some kind of retri-
bution. Parents who abandon their children really deserve to
be punished for what they've done.

Her therapist's nonjudgmental exploration of Ms. V's fears enabled this
patient to acknowledge intense aggression about which she was actually quite
afraid. Ms. V was terrified that if others saw her as angry, they would also
leave, as her father had left her and her embittered mother. Helping Ms. V to
acknowledge this fear was a crucial step toward working with this patient regarding her guilt, as well as her aggressive feelings toward her abandoning
parent. This understanding was a step toward her becoming more assertive
in expressing her needs and longings in her current relationships.

Identifying Expectations of Punishment

Many patients feel they will be punished for their aggressive, guilt-laden feelings. The fantasized punishments often take the form of rejection or attack by
others and often reflect the actual, vengeful ideas imagined by patients toward others, now turned against themselves. Castration, represented as being
disempowered in some fashion, may be perceived as a particularly distressing
danger, along with being unloved, rejected, or ridiculed.

Case Example 1C

As treatment progressed, further history emerged about Mr. T's experiences with women, shedding additional light on his guilty feelings. This
was his second marriage, and he had left his first wife for a much younger
woman about whom he felt more excited and passionate. Mr. T still felt
badly about this, and it seemed to him that his current wife's inattention was
a fitting punishment for this past behavior. This was represented in a dream
in which Mr. T learned his left hand would have to be amputated. The doctor in the dream said to him, underscoring his fantasies, "Well, you're old.
You won't be needing it anymore."

The dream also suggested that castration was another punishment that Mr. T was anticipating. In a sense, this was already occurring to the degree that he accepted the lack of sexual activity with his wife. He also felt castrated in the work setting: he felt his colleagues were getting perks he had once received regularly. Again, his fantasies indicated that he experienced this as a punishment as well and that his need for punishment to assuage his guilt was inhibiting him from taking steps that would allow him to make changes in his relationships.

Exploring the Link Between Competitiveness and Aggression

Because depressed patients have a history of intensified aggression connected to their early narcissistic injuries, they often become sensitized to and guilty about any aggressive impulses and work hard to inhibit them. Many depressed patients specifically link competitive wishes with their preexisting aggressive fantasies. Therefore, competitive feelings are prone to cause the same kind of guilt and self-recriminations as angry feelings and fantasies. Further, competitive fantasies are often linked with wishes for damage to and destruction of a rival. For depressed patients, such fantasies are particularly compelling, in that they may play a part in internal efforts to obtain more love and attention as a way of healing narcissistic wounds.

The earliest and most competitive feelings Mr. T recalled were aroused in regard to his older brother. He was angry that his brother was favored, particularly given his problematic and aggressive behavior. Efforts to compete with his brother were thwarted by the parents, who, however, did not intervene with his brother's bullying behavior. Mr. T later struggled with guilty feelings about being competitive with his colleagues in the work setting.

Case Example 1D

> MR. T: I know that in my efforts at work, I was trying to outdo my brother and show my parents they were wrong.
> THERAPIST: How did you feel about this?
> MR. T: Well, okay at first, but now I feel bad about it. I mean, I didn't expect things to go so badly for him. I hope I didn't cause any of it.
> THERAPIST: How would you have done that?
> MR. T: I guess by making him feel bad through doing well myself. Maybe I deserve the problems I'm having now.

THERAPIST: As punishment for your outdoing him?
MR. T: Yes, in a way.

Mr. T began to realize how much his difficulties in competing were linked with angry feelings that triggered guilt and a need for punishment. Thus, Mr. T did not take advantage of certain opportunities to expand his territories and be promoted when younger because he feared creating a conflict and felt guilty about his efforts to outdo his rivals. For similar reasons, he did not bring up certain creative ideas he had with his boss. Understanding these issues led to his feeling increased freedom to be assertive in his office as he felt safer with his competitive wishes. He had a dream in which his rival at work was having difficulty and he felt very happy about it, making him more aware and tolerant of the knowledge that he actually enjoyed outdoing others.

Becoming More Comfortable With Assertiveness

As patients feel safer with their angry feelings, they typically become more assertive in their daily lives. This can allow for a shift in some of the problematic aspects of their relationships that served to maintain their depression.

Case Example 1E

As described earlier, Mr. T wanted to confront his wife about her infrequent desire for sex but was inhibited by fears of disrupting their relationship further and by his feeling that he did not deserve more from her. Mr. T also experienced inadequacy with his therapist, fearing that the clinician wanted him to be more assertive with his wife and that he wasn't getting a "good grade" and was disappointing him. The therapist explored Mr. T's need to be the good patient and submit to what he felt the therapist required of him, just as he had with his mother to be the good little boy.

Mr. T then reported a dream in which his mother asked him whether her hair looked attractive. In the dream, Mr. T refused to respond to the question. Mr. T saw this dream as representing his newfound unwillingness to yield to demands of others. He had felt particularly relieved by being able to discuss the pressures he felt from the therapist.

After the exploration of this dream and of his perceived expectations of the therapist, Mr. T was finally able to confront his wife about their difficulties.

MR. T: I asked her whether she believed in monogamy. She was somewhat evasive. I told her that I would be very upset about the idea of her getting involved again with another man.

THERAPIST: And how did she respond to that?

MR. T: She didn't respond directly at the time, but since then, she's been quite solicitous and warmer.

THERAPIST: So confronting her didn't bring the results that you feared.

MR. T: No. I guess it was the opposite.

Mr. T's additional confrontations with his wife were also effective. There was an improvement in their sexual relationship, which seemed to become more passionate and expressive. This enabled the therapist to address Mr. T's previous perceptions of powerlessness and his shifting views of himself in relation to others.

THERAPIST: You've tended to see your wife as having all the power, while you needed to follow along because of your inadequacies. But it seems as if things look different to you now.

MR. T: I guess so. I've had more impact on her than I thought I could.

THERAPIST: Rather than being powerless, you actually have a power that you never suspected with her.

MR. T: Yes. I really wish I had seen that before. I was so worried that I no longer could have any impact in our relationship.

Mr. T's case followed the core dynamic of depression (depression cycle 1) in which narcissistic injuries experienced in childhood led to anger and vengeful fantasies of retaliating against loved ones to get what he needed. He felt guilty about these fantasies, further lowering his self-esteem, and feared punishment via castration or some other retaliation. Understanding these dynamics helped to reduce his guilt and allow for a more assertive stance at work and home that also relieved his feelings of inadequacy.

Recognizing Anger Directed Toward the Self

As angry feelings are experienced as potentially destructive, they frequently are directed toward the self to ease guilt and avert perceived damage to relationships. Other mechanisms that have been suggested for this self-direction of aggression include identification with the hated, rejecting, or lost other and negative reactions toward any aspect of the self that is seen as similar to the hated other (see Chapter 2). The therapist helps patients identify these self-attacks and aids them in recognizing their severity and lack of a realistic basis. The therapist then explores with patients the meanings

of these self-criticisms, with a focus on how the criticisms may represent angry attacks toward those by whom patients feel rejected, in the recent and
distant past. In addition, the therapist explores attacks on parts of the self that
patients identify with the rejecting other.

Case Example 4

Mr. W, a 48-year-old married lawyer in private practice presented with
several years of dysthymic symptoms. He complained about his marriage,
in which he felt that his wife was not adequately responsive to him sexually
and was "too negative." He was frustrated about his job, in which he experienced himself as underachieving and beset by forces beyond his control. He felt that he was a "nice guy" to his clients and his staff, making
him susceptible to being taken advantage of by his employees and feeling
deeply hurt if one of his clients left his practice. He would become preoccupied with anger at these people, ruminating about how to express these
feelings, while also feeling terribly guilty about them. For instance, he
would contemplate threatening his employees with dismissal if they did
not follow his edicts but would feel guilty and fear that they would quit. He
would then blame himself, saying that they only behaved this way because
he allowed it by not setting expectations for others. His therapist helped
Mr. W identify this pattern of anger at others being turned toward himself.

Mr. W viewed his family, particularly his mother, as having an agenda for
him that had little to do with his interests. He complained that when he was
a child, his mother took his toy gun away unfairly when another child complained to her about it, and that this exemplified her willingness to listen to
others while failing to consider his own happiness. When Mr. W wanted to
pursue architecture as a profession, his mother threatened to no longer speak
with him, insisting that he become a lawyer instead. Mr. W therefore experienced her as consistently withdrawing her love if he disagreed with her. His father was a more benign figure but, sadly, was minimally involved with his son.

Mr. W also revealed that his parents had rigid and strict rules about his
behavior, such as curfews. They would become very angry and ground him
when he came in late, even when there was a problem beyond his control.
He was infuriated that they would never listen to any of his explanations,
and he remembered banging his hand into a wall more than once after a
fight with his parents.

In attempting to set limits with his staff or expressing anger at others who
disappointed him, it emerged that Mr. W felt very much as if he were behaving in the rigid, hurtful way that his parents did. In addition, he experienced himself as threatening to "withdraw his love," just as he felt his mother
had with him. He would therefore see his behavior as terribly damaging to
others and feel guilty, fearing immediate rejection if he confronted them.

Mired in his conflicts about confronting others with his anger, Mr. W
generally directed anger toward himself via self-destructive behavior. For

instance, he would not exercise and he chain-smoked cigarettes. In addition, he would not be assertive in his career, and his law practice suffered.

The therapist and Mr. W came to recognize that he expressed his anger toward himself in exactly the ways that he wanted to express it to others. For instance, by failing at his career, he seemed to be telling his parents: "I'll do what you want, but I'm going to screw it up." His damage to his body appeared to represent the damage he wished to do to his parents, such as when he banged his hand into the wall in frustration. Recognizing that he was damaging himself to get back at his parents helped Mr. W to redirect his anger and reduce his self-destructive behaviors. Understanding that his anger was unlikely to create the same experience of damage among his employees that he had felt with his parents allowed Mr. W to begin to confront others appropriately.

Case Example 5

Ms. X, a 64-year-old housewife and mother of three, presented with a major depression, as well as with symptoms of chronically feeling ignored or attacked that were present prior to the onset of her current affective illness. Ms. X felt often very excluded by her husband, whom she experienced as having little empathy for her feelings, and as frequently placing financial concerns above their relationship. For instance, he had recently insisted on discussing with her his plans for their money if she were to die and he remarried, speaking about it in a way that she found hurtful and insensitive. She felt that he rarely talked to her but that he was very talkative with his friends. In addition, Ms. X felt often on the defensive against attacks by others in her life. This group included her brother, whom she viewed as very competitive with her, and her coworkers, whom she saw as derisive of her and others and as arrogant.

Ms. X recalled that her mother "couldn't stand her" and was very strict and critical, administering frequent spankings with a belt for minor infractions. Her mother did not tolerate any expressions of anger on the patient's part. Her father was a more affectionate and benign figure. She contrasted her husband with her father and found him wanting both emotionally and in his ambitions.

Ms. X was clearly very angry at her husband and her coworkers yet spent most of her time focusing on her anger at herself. She criticized herself for not accomplishing enough at work and at home and for not having enough friends. The therapist explored these tendencies.

THERAPIST: It really seems as if you are critical of everything about yourself.

MS. X: I guess I feel like I don't do much right.

THERAPIST: It sounds a lot like what your mother would tell you!

Ms. X: That's certainly true. It was terrible the way she treated me.

THERAPIST: But unlike her, you don't seem to talk directly to others about being angry at them.

Ms. X: Well, that's the thing. I was always told I'm not supposed to get angry. That's not okay.

THERAPIST: It seems like you then end up directing it at yourself. Is it okay to be brutal toward yourself?

Ms. X: I guess it is very harsh. Well, I don't want to turn it on others. I don't know what I would say to the women at work if I let my anger out, but it would be pretty bad.

THERAPIST: Well, I think we need to explore this anger further, but directing it at yourself takes a heavy toll.

Ms. X: I know. I feel in so much pain.

Working with these issues over time, Ms. X had a significant reduction in her self-attacks and began to experience improved relationships with her co-workers and friends. She had previously tended to withdraw from others, such as by not returning their phone calls, because she expected rejection. Then she felt rejected when they, in turn, stopped calling her. She changed this pattern by maintaining more regular contact with them. However, a few months after the death of her elderly mother, she had a resurgence in her depressive symptoms and self-attacks. This occurred after she had completed work on her mother's financial affairs and had planned a memorial for her. Ms. X was able to now acknowledge her anger at her mother, although she still seemed to struggle with guilt about this. Aware that this might be the case, the therapist urged Ms. X to continue to explore her current feelings about her mother.

Ms. X: I guess it's hard to believe that as nasty and hurtful as she was, I still miss having her around.

THERAPIST: I wonder if your constant criticisms of yourself are a way of keeping her with you, especially now that you've completed work on her affairs.

Ms. X: I guess it's possible. I mean, that was basically the whole of our relationship: her attacking me.

THERAPIST: And yet in many ways you remained very attached.

Ms. X: That's very true.

The realization that she missed her mother, despite her resentment of mistreatment by her mother, helped to ease Ms. X's recurrence of depression and paved the way for further mourning to take place. The therapist in part was employing Freud's (1917) view of melancholia versus mourning, with the patient internalizing her mother as a way of maintaining attachment and expressing the anger at her mother toward herself.

Case Example 6

Ms. Y was a 26-year-old single mother of one and a secretary who still lived with her parents. She reported a stream of intense criticism during her childhood, and even currently, from her father. She felt terribly injured and self-critical whenever her father berated her, even though she knew that what he said was often wrong or unfair. Once Ms. Y became somewhat comfortable in treatment, she reported worries that she would eventually reveal something bad inside herself to the therapist and that he would not want to be with her anymore. This patient also described her tendency to become involved in relationships in which her feelings were not returned.

> MS. Y [*describing an incident from the prior day*]: I left out the rest of the steak I had cooked, and the dog was licking it. All of a sudden my father was furious with me: "How could you leave it out like that? Now the meat is ruined. Go put it away."
>
> THERAPIST: And how did you feel?
>
> MS. Y: Well, I was down on myself for hours. I felt I had really screwed up. I felt inadequate and humiliated. With anyone else I would have just said, "Shut up and put the meat away if you want. I don't care if the dog licks it!"
>
> THERAPIST: You sound very angry when you describe how you would respond to someone else, but you have such a hard time getting angry with him!
>
> MS. Y: I hadn't really thought about it. I guess I am furious at him. But if I said anything, it would just lead to a fight. He would get more and more antagonistic. I'd lose.
>
> THERAPIST: It seems as if you then end up turning the anger on yourself.
>
> MS. Y: Yes. It seems that way. I guess it has to go somewhere.

During the next session, Ms. Y reported a dream: Her dogs were being very noisy and distracting. She screamed at them and then left the house.

> THERAPIST: What comes to mind about that dream?
>
> MS. Y: Well, I used to have a dog I would scream at all the time. I always felt really guilty about that.
>
> THERAPIST: The dogs remind me of how you described your father: distracting you and creating a lot of problems. Maybe you feel like screaming at him just like that.
>
> MS. Y: Yes. That's true. But I feel really guilty when I get so mad like that. I guess it's behaving like he does toward me. I know how much it hurts. I hate to do it.
>
> THERAPIST: Yes. And I think at times this keeps you from recognizing just how angry you are at someone, especially your fa-

ther. It's hard for you to realize at those times that there are
ways of confronting others that are not as hurtful as the way
your father does it.

Ms. Y: I think that's true. I need to learn better how to keep in
touch with these feelings.

In the cases discussed in this chapter, exploring the patients' self-directed
anger was of help in easing their depression. The realization that they were
attacking themselves with anger actually meant for someone else was of value
in easing their self-attacks. Understanding that they identified themselves,
when angry, with someone whom they experienced as hurtful, also helped
them to grapple with their conflicts. It was important for these patients to
understand the specific content of their anger and to develop more effective means of coping with it, such as by becoming more assertive with others with whom they were having difficulties, without fearing that they had
become rejecting or impossible themselves.

References

Abraham K: Notes on the psycho-analytical investigation and treatment of manic-
    depressive insanity and allied conditions (1911), in Selected Papers on Psycho-
    analysis. London, Hogarth Press, 1927, pp 137–156

Abraham K: A short study of the development of the libido, viewed in the light of
    mental disorders (1924), in Selected Papers on Psychoanalysis. London, Hogarth
    Press, 1927, pp 418–501

Freud S: Mourning and melancholia (1917), in The Standard Edition of the Com-
    plete Psychological Works of Sigmund Freud, Vol 14. Translated and edited
    by Strachey J. London, Hogarth Press, 1957, pp 239–258

Jacobson E: Depression: Comparative Studies of Normal, Neurotic, and Psychotic
    Conditions. New York, International Universities Press, 1971

Rado S: The problem of melancholia. Int J Psychoanal 9:420–438, 1928

Stone L: Psychoanalytic observations on the pathology of depressive illness: selected
    spheres of ambiguity or disagreement. J Am Psychoanal Assoc 34(2):329–362,
    1986 3722700

8

CHAPTER

The Severe Superego and Guilt

ALONG with narcissistic vulnerability and related affects of shame, help-lessness, and reactive anger, conscious or unconscious guilt often cripples de-pressed patients. Some patients reveal deep-seated feelings that they are bad or unworthy and are prone to attacking themselves—through self-criticisms or punishments—when they sense that they are behaving in an aggressive, com-petitive, or overly sexual manner. Examples of this are the cases of Ms. G in Chapters 4 ("Getting Started With Psychodynamic Treatment of Depression") and 6 ("Addressing Narcissistic Vulnerability"), who felt devastatingly guilty about aggressive thoughts concerning her mother and boyfriend, and of Ms. V in Chapter 7 ("Addressing Angry Reactions to Narcissistic Injury"), who wor-ried that she was harsh when expressing vindictive feelings toward her father.

Other patients seem to be unaware of guilty feelings, yet the therapist may infer them from these patients' self-punishing behaviors or self-criticisms. Some of these patients at times feel justified in their anger at their parents or others but experience unconscious conflict about some of their aggressive feelings and fantasies. As described below in this chapter (see the case of Ms. AA in Case Example 2), the therapist must be tactful in bringing evi-dence of unconscious guilt to patients' attention.

To best understand the depressive patient's guilt, it is important to review the theoretical concept of a harsh, or overly severe, superego (Arlow 1996). This concept is clinically useful in understanding patients who experience an uncontrollable inner sense of condemnation, those who experience no

Table 8–1.   Functions of the superego

1. *Judging:* Evaluating thoughts, desires, and fantasies as acceptable or harmful; can induce guilt

2. *Limiting:* Contains or limits impulses; inhibits behaviors

3. *Punitive or rewarding:* Punishes or praises the self, often by way of affects of guilt and depression or pleasure and pride

conscious guilt and whose self-punishment is only inferred, and those whose guilty feelings emerge in the course of psychotherapeutic exploration.

The superego is seen by some psychoanalysts (e.g., Milrod 1972) as a complex inner structure having three functions (Table 8–1): 1) a judging function, which evaluates behaviors, thoughts, desires, and even fantasies as either acceptable or as morally harmful to the self or to others and which can often stimulate the conscious experience of guilt; 2) a limiting function, which contains or limits impulses and inhibits behaviors judged to be unacceptable; and 3) a punitive or rewarding function, which is responsible for actually punishing a patient for unacceptable thoughts or impulses or rewarding praiseworthy actions. Punishment can occur in the form of tormenting guilt or other depressive affects or can be accomplished by way of stimulating self-destructive behaviors. Often the self-punitive aspect or guilty trigger of these behaviors occurs outside of the patient's awareness or is only minimally understood.

Severity in the superego can have many different etiologies, as decribed in part in Chapter 2 ("Development of a Psychodynamic Model of Depression"). For example (see discussion about Ms. AA in Case Example 2), a harsh, judging superego can be based, at least partly, on internalizing the accusations of a parent perceived as excessively punitive, blaming, or demanding. Some depressed patients, however, have had parents who were experienced as neglectful, frustrating, or even overindulgent rather than harsh. These patients may fear that aggressive fantasies toward frustrating, withdrawn, or neglectful parents could get out of control and damage them, stimulating the development of a harsh, limiting superego. Further, hostile or competitive impulses toward parents who are perceived as psychologically or physically fragile can stimulate an excessive sense of guilt, through the fear that one can, or even has, damaged this parent. Patients whose parents are overindulgent may have the fantasy that they might "get away with murder," triggering guilt and conflict. In these various instances, the development of a harsh and limiting superego can result in a compensatory, excessive inner scrutiny, an excessive limitation of consciously experienced aggressive or

---

Table 8–2.   Working with the harsh superego: middle phase of treatment

---

1.   Helping patients recognize hidden guilt and self-punishment in their behaviors and feelings
2.   Exploring guilt-laden fantasies
3.   Identifying anger, guilt, and self-punishment embedded in character: severe inhibitions and sadomasochistic character traits

---

sexual wishes, and an inhibition of behaviors and thoughts that are unconsciously linked to these fantasies.

In working with depressed patients, then, understanding and interpreting the different functions of a harsh superego can contribute to alleviating conscious and unconscious guilt, to diminishing self-punishment expressed through destructive behaviors and tormenting depressive affects, and to relieving excessive inhibitions based on guilt and on an excessively limiting superego (Table 8–2). The latter outcome, in turn, allows patients greater opportunity for self-expression and for behaviors that will enhance their self-esteem and diminish feelings of narcissistic vulnerability.

Helping Patients Recognize Guilt and Self-Punishment

In working with patients who experience little conscious guilt, it is sometimes difficult to help them to become aware of this dimension of their dynamics. Invariably, however, they display self-punitive affects or behaviors from which an attuned observer might infer a guilty self-appraisal. It is important to help patients become aware of their unconscious guilt and consequent self-punishment. It is often useful to start with an exploration of the self-punishing feelings and behaviors themselves. For some patients, examining the temporal course of these feelings and behaviors is quite illuminating, especially because depressed individuals often punish themselves for positive developments in their lives of which they feel unworthy or which they may interpret as resulting from unacceptably aggressive or sexual behaviors (Brenner 1975, 1979) (see Chapter 2).

Case Example 1

Ms. Z was a 24-year-old artist who had become immobilized after her first show garnered very favorable reviews. In the months that followed, she became progressively unable to work at her art, lying on her couch and watching television for much of the day, taking up smoking, and hating herself thoroughly for her sense of paralysis. Ms. Z felt numb and, on occasion, unpredictably tearful. But she was unaware of any guilty feelings, except for self-criticisms about being "lazy; I'm a complete slug!," which she felt were entirely justified, given her current behavior. It was only when her behavior alarmed her boyfriend, and he was insistent, that Ms. Z sought treatment.

Initial work with Ms. Z aimed at helping her understand her current behavior as guilty and intensely self-punishing. This was accomplished by linking it with aspects of her history about which she was more self-aware.

> MS. Z: I feel like an idiot that I didn't recognize that this was a depression. I just sort of drifted into it. But I have been depressed before, and the same thing happened. I don't think I realized it until later, then, either. And my parents just didn't seem to get it at all, that I was profoundly unhappy.
> THERAPIST: Can you tell me about that time?
> MS. Z: It was after my rape, at age 14.

This young woman had gone to a party with some older neighborhood friends during the fall of her freshman year in high school. Not used to drinking alcohol, she had become intoxicated, and in this state, as she looked for her coat to leave the party, found herself in a bedroom with three boys. At first amused and surprised by their flirtatious behavior, she became frightened when their mood turned ugly and they virtually forced her to perform fellatio on one of them. She half protested, half submissively participated, then ran away from the party, vomiting and feeling violated and ashamed. She told no one about the episode, but her behavior changed abruptly. Previously a "good girl" at school, she now seemed driven to be "bad": for the first time, she actively and promiscuously sought out sexual contacts, became inattentive to and had great difficulty concentrating on her studies, and felt miserable, anhedonic, and self-hating for months.

> MS. Z [tearful]: It was like an orgy of bad feelings about myself. My parents just made it worse by yelling at me. I guess I wasn't surprised that they yelled; I felt so awful about myself.
> THERAPIST: It really does sound as if the same kind of thing is happening now, don't you think? You did get your boyfriend very worried about you.
> MS. Z: Yes, but he had the sense to tell me to see a therapist. My parents just flailed around.
> THERAPIST: It sounds like you blamed yourself terribly for what happened to you then.
> MS. Z: I think so. I was so innocent, and wham! What might have been a funny kind of story to tell your friends changed into something so awful.

THERAPIST: You were drunk and trying out what it felt like to flirt with some boys. When it escalated, you thought you made it happen that way.

MS. Z: Yes. It wasn't until years later that I even realized how furious I was with those guys. At the time, I felt I did something dumb and foolish—gave the wrong kind of signals—and... wham!

After reviewing the past episode of depression, in which the link between guilt and self-punishment is clear, the therapist turned toward the present:

THERAPIST: And now—let's try to understand what is happening now. You had a successful show, with really good reviews, and the next thing you know...

MS. Z: I can't function.

THERAPIST: Absolutely. I think that what is happening now connects to those events from the past. There you were, trying to flirt with these boys who seemed interested in you, and they behaved so cruelly...as if punishing you for responding to them. Maybe now you still connect efforts to feel sexy, assertive, and self-expressive with punishment. After the rape, you punished *yourself* by your self-destructive behavior, and you are doing the same thing now. This time, it is for showing the world who you are, expressing yourself in your show, even being playful and sexy in some of your artwork.

Somewhat later in this treatment, as therapist and patient explored more of Ms. Z's family life, they discovered predispositions to her reactions to these boys at age 14. Ms. Z's mother was a bright, self-denying woman who had left college early because she had become pregnant with Ms. Z's older brother. Many covert and some explicit messages within her family signaled that trying to get ahead would be met with frustration and punishment and that sexuality was a dangerous business. When Ms. Z encountered these boys, she was primed to interpret their behavior as a swift punishment for her experiment at flirtation. Her judging and punitive superego functions were quite harsh.

Case Example 2

Ms. AA, a 45-year-old real estate broker, had a relapse of depression and anxiety during psychotherapy. Normally an ebullient woman with many friends with whom she enjoyed socializing, she withdrew, canceled appointments with her clients and therapist, and remained at home, sleeping through the mornings, overeating and feeling miserable and anxious. Such symptoms, if persistent, would lead to a consideration of medication intervention as well as psychotherapy (see Chapter 15 "Use of Psychodynamic Psychotherapy With Other Treatment Approaches").

Her therapist elected to trace the depressed behavior in time, in order to understand its precursors.

THERAPIST: You seemed to be doing well when we met 10 days ago. Do you remember when it was that you started feeling so depressed?

MS. AA: No, but I just have to get rid of these feelings. It's terrible.

THERAPIST: Okay; let's try to understand what might have provoked them. What do you remember was happening when you started feeling this way?

MS. AA [*thoughtful*]: I guess I understand something about this, but it all seems so trivial. I was talking to my neighbor Selena last week, and she was very upset with our other neighbor, Anne. Anne has always been nice to me, but Selena was describing ways in which she can be really awful; she always snubs her. It was a real eye-opener, and I found myself getting really angry, putting it together with other gossipy things Anne has said to me about other people. I felt so bad for Selena and so angry at Anne. And then, as we were talking, Anne came outside to pick up her mail. She saw us talking. I know it's foolish to think this, but I thought she might have understood that we were talking about her.

THERAPIST: And how did you react to that thought?

MS. AA: I felt really anxious. I thought that now Anne will dislike me and make my life miserable in our neighborhood. I started thinking that we should consider moving. I know that's silly. But I felt right in the middle of a big fight, and it was awful. I have avoided Anne and also Selena ever since.

THERAPIST: It sounds as if Anne suddenly became kind of a monster in your eyes.

MS. AA: Yes, it scared me so much that she might know how angry I was just then. I know this is probably all exaggerated, but I feel so awful about it. I still feel sympathetic with Selena, and I think Anne probably is a mean person.

THERAPIST: A mean person who will punish you and take revenge at you for feeling so angry. You are *very* anxious about that. But I think that there is more here to understand than the anxiety and the way it makes you avoid both women. We need to understand why you are also so depressed.

MS. AA: I guess that thinking about Anne being mean must have triggered the feelings I always have about my mother. It made

me feel helpless, like "Oh, no, here it is all over again. I'm living with another awful person and I can't deal with it."

Ms. AA had discussed her relationship with her mother extensively in
this treatment. Her mother was described as a paranoid woman who had
attacked her daughter viciously and unpredictably at times, both verbally
and physically. Ms. AA was terrified of her and often became anxious in
situations when she was exposed to angry women, especially older women.
She was aware of her anger toward her mother, insisting it was justified,
and experienced little guilt about it. This seemed an opportune time to
help Ms. AA recognize not only the helplessness and accompanying sense
of intense vulnerability that she was experiencing in her depression but
also the guilt for her rageful feelings.

> THERAPIST: Exactly! I do think the depression is coming from a sense
> of helplessness that is really familiar to you. But there is also the
> fact of your anger—you're convinced that Anne will punish
> you for it. I think that this depression is a way of punishing
> *yourself* first—maybe then no one will punish you, when they
> see how helpless you are. I also think that even though your an-
> ger may be justified, being angry makes part of you feel like a
> bad person. You are punishing yourself for that, for being bad.
> MS. AA: Hmm…well, that does make sense, I guess. If I punish
> myself first, maybe no one else will have to. But you make it
> seem as if I *am doing something to myself* when I'm depressed,
> not just that I am so helpless. I'm not sure I like that idea.
> I feel so helpless, like something has just come over me, when
> I'm this sad. It doesn't feel as if I'm doing this to myself at all!

This is a common objection to the idea that depression is, in part, a
form of self-punishment. Although depressive affects can be stimulated by
fantasies about rejection, damage, or helplessness, the self-torment of the
depressive state is often connected to fantasies about guilt and wrong-doing.
This patient felt most comfortable with interpretations about her helplessness in the relationship with her disturbed mother. Ms. AA was aware that
she was deeply angry with her mother but felt consciously that her rage was
justified. It was important for her to see that despite this conscious feeling
of entitlement to her anger, that she was also unconsciously guilty. Introducing the idea of a harsh conscience, or superego, can be helpful in addressing
this difficulty, as follows:

> THERAPIST: Well, I do think that *one part of you*, your conscience,
> *is attacking* another part of yourself. Sometimes our con-

science isn't very rational. It *was* shaped by our earliest experiences and sometimes can be very *irrational.* Maybe part of you took in what your mother said about you when she was being so mean, and deep down, you really *do* feel like an angry, bad person.

Ms. AA: Hmm…I did feel pretty bad sometimes as a kid. It just felt so oppressive, those things my mother said, and it makes sense that of course, I believed them. It just seems as if I should be over that. But maybe you're right. Maybe part of me still believes all that.…And maybe part of me is also trying to control what the other person thinks. Like—I'm saying, "I'm not a threat! I'm not bad! I'm just a lump of anxiety and sadness. Stay away!"

The image of the judging superego, based on internalizing her mother's accusations, helped Ms. AA to see that she had guilty fantasies, outside of her awareness, about what she consciously viewed as justifiable rage. The vignette presents another important aspect of psychological functioning, in that individuals can have different representations of self and others sometimes operating at odds and unrecognized. For instance, someone could be fluctuating between submission and rebellion or, as in the vignette, anger and guilty self-punishment. Making these various aspects of self and other representations conscious is crucial to increased understanding and integration of the self and relief of symptoms.

Exploring Guilt-Laden Fantasies

Once patients recognize that they may be feeling guilty and punishing themselves with depressive symptoms, it is important to explore the fantasies that might be triggering the guilt. For Ms. Z, succeeding in the art world meant that she was surpassing her mother, whose life was extremely frustrating, as well as her sister, who had many physical and emotional difficulties. Ms. Z's mother, in fact, had often suggested to the patient that her good looks and talent made her younger sister feel bad. She had come to connect self-expression, especially expressions of her sexuality, with punishment. Ms. AA, on the other hand, seemed to have internalized a sense of herself, especially when she was angry, as being bad and deserving of attack, either from others or from herself. This sense seems to have been formed in the context of her relationship with her rather disturbed, vindictive mother, who often accused the patient of being bad, highly destructive, and sinful.

Looking for evidence that patients have internal fantasies of being bad or unworthy or feel guilty about fantasies connected with sexuality, aggression, or autonomy is helpful for those individuals who recognize their guilt but are confused about its source. Many patients imagine, rather concretely, that they are punishing themselves for some specific action made during childhood. They may need help in understanding that guilt and punishment do not always attach to one specific, possibly secret deed but rather to a range of feelings and ideas about oneself and one's actions that have accumulated over time and in the context of ongoing relationships with important others.

Case Example 3

Mr. BB, a much-loved 50-year-old teacher in a prestigious private school, was often troubled by gnawing feelings of guilt, especially in the context of his relationship with his wife, in which he felt unable to meet her needs. These guilty feelings seemed embedded in Mr. BB's character and occurred frequently. When he was clinically depressed, which had occurred on three occasions in his life, Mr. BB's sense of guilt became paralyzing.

In his treatment, therapist and patient had identified a crucial time in Mr. BB's childhood when his mother had become depressed and he had felt sad and frightened by her emotional unavailability. She had been markedly withdrawn, in contrast to her usual caring demeanor. Mr. BB had been especially dependent on his mother, as his father seemed a rather insolent, sullen man who resented having to share his wife's attention. His therapist thought it likely that Mr. BB's guilty self-recriminations were multiply determined and must have been set in motion, at least partly, by rage over his father's disappointing immaturity and his lack of attention to the patient. However, the therapist also suspected, given Mr. BB's sense of utter responsibility in the present, that Mr. BB might have felt responsible, too, for his mother's depression. This remained a theoretical speculation, however, until the following exchange occurred. In the course of a session, Mr. BB had mentioned his unhappiness at having to spend time after school being cared for by his aunt, with whom he did not get along.

> THERAPIST: I don't recall that we've talked about this before. Can you tell me more about it? What didn't you like about being with her?
>
> MR. BB: What didn't I like? Everything! I realized later that she was an alcoholic. I certainly don't remember any outrageous or drunken behavior during those afternoons, but it did always seem as if…things were just so much less organized in her home. It was very boring. Everyone just drifted around watching TV. I didn't have anything in common with my

cousins, and I just felt very different from all of them. They were angry kids, too—sometimes my uncle would be home and he would beat them over something they did. He never touched *me*, but I was scared. I think they resented that I was treated differently, and sometimes they would take that out on me....

THERAPIST: Did you ever tell your mother how bad you felt about being there?

MR. BB: I did, in my own way. But she had to work, and I think she felt that it was important that I have a connection to our wider family since my family is so small—just the three of us. Looking back, I think I kind of just expected that she would know what it was like, and she probably really didn't at all.

Because Mr. BB had such difficulty recognizing and discussing angry feelings toward anyone, his therapist made an effort to elicit these, making an indirect point that such feelings toward his mother would be natural in this situation.

THERAPIST: So you told her in your own way, thinking that she would understand, but she really didn't. I wonder if that didn't make you upset with her.

MR. BB: I don't think so....But even if I were upset, where would that leave me? We couldn't really easily make any other arrangements, and I didn't want to make her unhappy....She was the one who generally did understand, you know. She was pretty wonderful, and I just didn't want to be angry with her.

As Mr. BB had not acknowledged being angry but did admit how difficult it would have been to have such feelings, the therapist directly and empathically described what she assumed was the patient's dilemma.

THERAPIST: That was quite a problem, though, for you, wasn't it? You loved her and maybe sensed her fragility, too. And you needed her—out of all these adults, she was the one who usually understood what you were going through. But you probably deep down also really missed her during those afternoons and blamed her for leaving you in this bad situation, in which you felt different from the others and vulnerable because of that.

MR. BB: I think it was always very hard to be angry with her, because I did need her and I loved her. I didn't ever want to add to her burdens at all.

The therapist then summarized the fantasies that she discerned the patient might have had in this context, and connected them to both his depression and to the chronic character inhibitions that made him vulnerable to sadness or shameful, self-accusatory affects.

> THERAPIST: So you felt bad about having any angry feelings, and you tried so hard not to need more than she could give you. I think, as a result, you have tended to feel *very* responsible for the people around you! That is a wonderful trait, but it also makes it hard for you to allow yourself any room to just enjoy things, without feeling selfish! It makes you torment yourself when the people you care about have problems. You feel as if you failed them and caused their troubles. I don't know if you blamed yourself for your mother's depression, but you do seem to have felt that you *could* cause her sadness or unhappiness, just by being upset with her or needing a bit more than she could give.
>
> MR. BB: I guess so. I can see in my marriage that I try very hard never to be upset with my wife, but I guess when you live with anyone, you will get angry from time to time. And when I am angry or resentful with her, I really get upset with myself. I feel: "Suck it up—why add to her troubles?"

In this vignette, the excessive sense of responsibility that made it difficult for Mr. BB to enjoy his life was seen as connected with an old set of fears and fantasies. Mr. BB had imagined that he would cause deep unhappiness in his mother if he spoke about his disappointment and anger, as exemplified when she left him in an unsuitable after-school environment. He gradually internalized his anger, felt inadequate that he was not happy in this situation and others, and redoubled his efforts to "be good" and care for his mother, whom he (likely accurately) perceived as rather fragile. This case represents an example of the development of a severe superego secondary to fears and guilt about potentially damaging a parent.

In his current situation, Mr. BB would punish himself by feeling ashamed and low if he thought that he was failing to keep up his role as a caring helper. Much of his treatment focused on helping Mr. BB realize that although he might have had reasons to be protective of his mother as a child, the guilt that he had experienced about feelings that had seemed disloyal or hurtful to her had been excessive. With these insights, as well as with additional work on guilt over angry feelings toward his father, Mr. BB was gradually able to allow himself a much greater flexibility and happiness in his adult life. This change may be viewed as resulting from increased self-acceptance in the judging aspect of his superego, a diminished harshness in its punitive function, and an acceptance of a wider range of allowable behavior in its limiting aspects.

Case Example 4

Mr. M, whose case was previously discussed in Chapter 5 (see Case Example 5 in that chapter), was a lawyer in his late-30s who had chronic dysthymia and major depression when he sought psychotherapy. He was unhappy in his marriage and highly judgmental about his work performance, which in fact did seem to be hampered by chronic inhibitions. In addition, he experienced anxiety and had begun having panic attacks. In his psychotherapy, Mr. M's anxiety and panic symptoms stabilized first. He realized how frightened he was of distancing others with his hostility, yet how often he experienced interpersonal interactions as freighted with conflict and a struggle for control.

It emerged that his mother had become ill with cancer when he was 13, dying 3 years later after several disfiguring surgical procedures. Prior to her illness, the two had struggled over Mr. M's wishes to become more independent, and these struggles had escalated with her failing health. His mother needed him to help out, and sometimes, when she interrupted him while he was outside playing sports, he would delay returning to assist her, causing angry altercations. As the therapy continued, it became clear that Mr. M had the fantasy that he had caused her death through his desire for independence and his angry outbursts when this was thwarted. His depression seemed to serve as a guilty punishment as well as a symbolic castration: he was rendered passive, unable to perform in an independent or assertive manner.

Further, Mr. M revealed that his father had been a passive man and that the family had gone into a downward spiral after his mother's death, having to sell their house and move to smaller quarters. Mr. M had been angry and disappointed in his father for his failures but was again fearful that his rage could overwhelm this man. In his adult life, the patient seemed to identify with his father's passivity and hold himself back as a way of protecting others from his aggression.

In his treatment, guilt over competitive, oedipally based feelings toward Mr. M's father emerged as well. As the patient was discussing a panic attack that occurred as he was shaving, his therapist noted that shaving was something that only men, and not boys, did. Mr. M instantly had a memory of an incident from his childhood, which he described as happening while he was in his own bathroom. Then, catching himself, the patient revealed that the event had actually taken place in his father's bathroom. Through examining this slip, therapist and patient came to realize that Mr. M imagined that he could be a competent and effective man only if he replaced or in some way negated his father. Because Mr. M perceived his father as rather fragile, these wishes and fantasies about replacing him made him very guilty, as if they actually had damaged his father.

Again, psychotherapeutic work elucidated Mr. M's guilt about aggressive feelings and behaviors that he imagined had damaged both parents. When he recognized that his guilt was based on unrealistic fantasies, it helped diminish his harsh self-judgment and relax his punitive and excessively limiting stance. As noted in Chapter 5, "The Middle Phase of Treatment," work was also done to address guilt about sexual feelings he had experienced toward his mother.

Identifying Anger, Guilt, and Self-Punishment Embedded in Character

Some depressed patients can seem, even to their therapists, to experience recurrences "out of the blue," apparently related to a biological susceptibility to that mood state. In such patients, reductions in medication can be a contributing factor to recurrences of their depressions. However, in our clinical experience, certain personality traits and vulnerabilities are also clearly implicated in a susceptibility to recurrences for most dysthymic and depressed patients. Even for patients who relapse as they are weaned off their medications, some predisposing features of their psychology may make them additionally vulnerable. The presence of a severe superego that limits pleasure and harshly judges or punishes anger, assertiveness, or sexuality is a major predisposing factor to chronic depression and to depressive relapses. It is thus important to recognize and to treat the kinds of self-punishing character adaptations that occur within patients in response to a harsh superego.

One such type of character adaptation, discussed by Asch (1988) in regard to its relationship to depression, is masochism. Masochism is a multi-determined phenomenon in which patients seem excessively predisposed to suffering. This predisposition may result partly from a severely limiting superego function, which inhibits and constricts most impulses, rendering the patient unable to enjoy the pleasures of sexuality or of self-assertion. Such was the case with Mr. BB, who blamed himself so excessively for any failures in his caretaking that his own experiences of pleasure were drastically curtailed. In more severe cases, one may sense that the only, or the predominant, pleasures afforded such a patient derive, in fact, from a sense of suffering. Further, not only can chronic suffering or feelings of victimization punish a person for fantasized wrongdoing but it can also provide a disguised outlet for aggression. Horowitz (1999) wrote about the pleasures of imagined vengeance at work in the dynamics of such patients, who subtly blame others while portraying themselves as blameless, helpless victims. An example might be a patient who attempts suicide in response to a rejection, with this act intended, at least partially, to provoke lifelong guilt in the rejecting party. Whether one detects the pleasure in pain, which is the hallmark of masochism, or simply the chronic suffering due to inhibition that dramatically curtails self-esteem, it is crucial to focus on these embedded character features that may predispose some depressed patients to dysthymia or to future depessive episodes.

As therapeutic work on the self-punishing inhibitions and self-destructive behaviors unfolds, one can see the connection between underlying masochism (or the tendency to self-punishment, sometimes secretly or unconsciously enjoyed) and hidden sadism (an enjoyment of vengeful fantasies and actions). These paired (sadomasochistic) tendencies can result in a chronic sense of shame and guilt, with flare-ups in depressive affects when they are exacerbated.

Case Example 5

Ms. CC, a 40-year-old translator, grew up in a war-torn country and experienced multiple traumas during her childhood. Sent away from her city as it was bombed when she was 4 years old, she was terrified that her parents would not survive. She remembered being confused about the reasons for her dislocation and disliking the distant relatives with whom she boarded. One of their sons tormented her unmercifully about her shy fearfulness and on occasion pushed or hit her. Shortly after Ms. CC finally rejoined her family, she was injured in an accident in which another child picked up a stray hand grenade, which exploded. She was disfigured by her injury.

Ms. CC realized in retrospect that both parents were "in shock" and quite depressed for some time after the war. There was little food available, and survival was a struggle. Life eventually stabilized, however, and Ms. CC, a bright girl, succeeded in school and went on to college. However, depression and a gradually evolving pattern of self-sabotage crippled her progress. Ms. CC became quite depressed shortly before her college graduation, dropped out, and, even after her depression abated, could not bring herself to complete her final courses. When she presented for treatment years later, she had drifted from one poorly paying translating job to another. She avoided relationships with men, except for brief affairs that left her yearning for more. During one of these, she became pregnant and continued the pregnancy but gave up her daughter for adoption. Several years later, on the anniversary of her daughter's birth, Ms. CC became profoundly depressed.

In therapy, it became apparent that Ms. CC linked her child's fate with her own wartime experience of abandonment. Her simmering guilt about the adoption had flared with the child's birthday and was exacerbated after Ms. CC read in the newspapers about another child whose adoptive parents had abused her.

MS. CC: I just can't believe that I gave up my child. I think that I did a terrible thing.
THERAPIST: Can you tell me what went into your decision? Were you feeling pressured by your family?

It is often tempting, with a patient who has experienced so much trauma, to try to "soften" things for them, the way that, for example, the therapist implied to Ms. CC that the decision was her parents' responsibility and not the patient's. However, rapidly offering ways to lessen guilt is generally to be avoided: guilty patients may seem to seek temporary dispensation or blame of others, but entrenched guilt is rarely helped, and is sometimes exacerbated, by such techniques. It is better to elicit information about the content of the patient's self-accusation and then work from there. Therapist and patient can then assess what is actually blameworthy, as compared with what is exaggerated, amplified, or projected because of the patient's internal fantasies.

MS. CC: To some extent, yes. They were ashamed, and also they did not believe that I could manage caring for a child. But I didn't think I could, either.
THERAPIST: Can you tell me about that?
MS. CC [*sobbing*]: I...really can't. I feel like such a bad person. But...I wasn't sure a child would be safe with me, either.
THERAPIST: You were afraid you might hurt the baby in some way?
MS. CC: I have had bad thoughts sometimes. They are very shameful. But now, I have cast this child out, away from its mother. And I remember how terrible I felt in that house, with that other family. I felt so alone.

As this treatment progressed, Ms. CC was gradually able to reveal fantasies that tormented her, in which she became sexually excited imagining children being beaten. She was greatly ashamed of these fantasies. Additionally, there had been a period during her childhood, after she recovered from her injury, in which she had kicked or thrown rocks at stray dogs. Ms. CC had been terrified that she might similarly hurt her daughter.

Her therapist suggested to Ms. CC that these fantasies and enactments were rooted in her tormented responses to her early traumas. In the sexual fantasies, Ms. CC was likely imagining turning the tables on the child in her temporary home who had tormented her. In her aggression against the animals, Ms. CC was perhaps identifying with him and with another powerful aggressor: the enemy whose bombs and weapons had torn apart her family and maimed her body.

Ms. CC gradually revealed her conviction that her wartime injury made her disgusting and unlovable. She felt that her daughter would have been repelled by her and was better off living with an "intact American family who had never suffered the way I have." On the other hand, she wrestled with her own disgust at and envy of Americans who had never experienced wartime. Ms. CC recognized, over time, that she secretly enjoyed putting down the naivete that she perceived in many of those now around her, and she realized that sometimes her acerbic humor made others uncomfortable. Although such put-downs made her feel temporarily superior, these would be quickly followed by brief periods of depression or by self-punishing behaviors, such as missing deadlines or smoking cigarettes with a vengeance.

Ms. CC also learned to distinguish between her suffering during her wartime dislocation and her child's very different situation. "I guess she really is having a very different experience. After all, she never knew me, so she wasn't wrenched away, like me, from everything she knew or cared about."

Ms. CC also gradually forgave herself for the aspects of her decision that represented an imagined identification with her parents' thoughts, as they sent her away. "I think I always felt that they were mean and punishing me for something bad that I did. Maybe part of me hated this baby for what I imagined she would eventually feel about me: that I was a bad person, ugly and damaged. And so I sent her off. But mostly, in reality, I think I made the right decision for her. Maybe one day I will try to find her, to see for myself."

Though Ms. CC continued to struggle at times with tormented thoughts and feelings, these insights gradually helped to resolve her depression. Her case demonstrates the importance of eliciting the specific fantasies that accompany guilty self-assessments and of empathically encouraging patients to discuss both sadistic as well as masochistic fantasies and enactments. This can be of enormous help in relieving the significant guilt and shame that accompany such fantasies. Through this kind of work, inhibitions can be gradually eased and tendencies toward self-punishment interrupted. For Ms. CC, the ability to express long-strangulated feelings of helplessness, confusion, and reactive hatred was tremendously helpful in her recovery from her depressive episode. She became better able to understand her actions and fantasies and to at least partly forgive, rather than continue to excoriate, herself for them.

References

Arlow J: The structural model, in Textbook of Psychoanalysis. Edited by Nersessian E, Kopff RG Jr. Washington, DC, American Psychiatric Press, 1996, pp 57–81

Asch S: The analytic concept of masochism: a re-evaluation, in Masochism: Current Clinical Perspectives. Edited by Glick R, Meyers D. Hillsdale, NJ, Analytic Press, 1988, pp 93–116

Brenner C: Affects and psychic conflict. Psychoanal Q 44(1):5–28, 1975 1114198

Brenner C: Depressive affect, anxiety, and psychic conflict in the phallic-oedipal phase. Psychoanal Q 48(2):177–197, 1979 441209

Horowitz M: On the difficulty of analyzing character. Journal of Clinical Psychoanalysis 8:212–217, 1999

Milrod D: Self-pity, self-comforting, and the superego. Psychoanal Study Child 27:505–528, 1972

9

CHAPTER

Idealization
and Devaluation

AS discussed in Chapter 8 ("The Severe Superego and Guilt"), depressed patients can have scrupulously held moral standards. Additionally, their personal expectations of themselves in other realms of endeavor can be unrealistic. These attitudes are rooted in an excessively perfectionistic ego ideal. The ego ideal, considered to be another dimension of the superego, establishes goals to be met and attributes to be held for the person to consider the self praiseworthy or deserving of respect. Failures to meet excessive expectations give rise to depressive affects of shame, humiliation, or unworthiness, as distinct from the guilt stimulated by a failure to meet moral standards.

Reich (1960) described self-esteem regulation as depending on the "nature of the inner image against which we measure our own self, as well as on the ways and means at our disposal to live up to it" (p. 216). Persons who are narcissistically vulnerable because of traumatic early experiences of helplessness, rejection, or loss often develop compensatory unconscious fantasies of power, magnificence, or invulnerability in themselves or in those on whom they depend. They may fluctuate between severe feelings of inadequacy and self-criticism alternating with compensatory grandiose self-views (Kohut 1971). Such fantasies and fluctuations interfere with the development of a realistic ego ideal or wished-for self-image (Milrod 1982) based on the actual or reasonable abilities of the individual. When the individual fails to meet such highly unrealistic expectations, depression may ensue or he or she looks to others to offset the resulting sense of diminishment.

Depressed individuals may search for mentors, friends, lovers, and therapists who appear to be "perfect," strong, and whole, with the magical hope that they will confer these qualities on the patient through their relationship. In fact, such patients may regain feelings of value through their identification with such an idealized individual or organization (see case of Ms. C in Chapter 2, "Development of a Psychodynamic Model of Depression"). Alternatively, they may devalue others to bolster their low self-esteem.

In the case of idealization, however, when the other person fails in some way to meet the depressed person's standards, trouble can result. Their relationship no longer confers the same sense of specialness, and the depressed individual, feeling again diminished, may scramble to protect the friend or loved one from his angry disappointment and, in the process, distort the reality of what has occurred. The depressed person may blame himself incorrectly or feel helpless about his ability to assess the situation accurately. Alternatively, he may reject the other person as devalued. The aggression in such a stand, however, can result in conscious or unconscious guilt, as discussed in Chapter 8, triggering depression. In this set of dynamics, depression cycle 2 (idealization/disappointment/loss of self-esteem) can trigger depression cycle 1 (anger/guilt/self-criticism/depression).

Just as fantasies of grandly overcoming helplessness, loss, or castration can shape an unrealistic wished-for self-image, so, too, may an internalization of unrealistic parental expectations and attitudes. For example, patients may feel a chronic sense of inadequacy about their failure to live up to expectations shaped by parents who were grandiose or unempathetic with their realistic difficulties.

Unrealistic cultural norms can result in a susceptibility for individuals within a group to feel pressured by the demanding standards of its shared ego ideal. Arieti and Bemporad (1978) discussed a study that contrasted the child-rearing practices of the neighboring Ojibwa and Eskimo tribes and linked these to their members' different susceptibilities to depression. Although they shared similar environmental hardships, these peoples conceptualized their relationship to the harsh conditions differently. Eskimo children were treated with patience, tolerance, and gratification, with expectations of joint work for community survival slowly introduced. Ojibwa children, on the other hand, were "toughened" to face difficult lives on their own, and regularly starved to prepare them for future periods of food shortages. It was expected that they would meet these demands without complaint.

The Ojibwa demonstrated a very high rate of depressive illness in contrast to their neighbors. Genetic factors could certainly play a role in this differ-

Table 9–1. Working with idealization and devaluation
1. Identifying idealization and devaluation of the self
2. Addressing idealization and devaluation of others
3. Exploring idealization and devaluation in the transference

ence. However, it seemed as if individuals within this group experienced both feelings of guilt and moral failure if they did not succeed on an individual basis, as well as feelings of shame and personal devaluation if they did not meet the unrealistic demands of their group's shared ego ideal. It is likely, from a psychoanalytic perspective, that this tendency toward devaluation was mediated by way of an internalization of the unrealistic group standard as well as individual fantasies about helplessness and compensatory power, stimulated by the unrealistic demands on individuals within this culture. We will discuss ways of addressing idealization and devaluation, including identifying idealization and devaluation of self and others, and exploring these elements in the transference (see Table 9–1).

Identifying Idealization and Devaluation of the Self

When patients strive relentlessly for perfection in order to feel less damaged or vulnerable and plummet into despair when they fail to achieve this idealized state, it is crucial to call their attention to the unrealistic nature of their self-assessments. As always, it is most helpful to discern the specific content of individual fantasies about perfection or failure.

Case Example 1

Ms. DD was the only daughter of parents whose marriage was strained throughout her early years. Her mother seemed to work long hours to escape her painful feelings about this relationship, and her father, often angry, was physically punitive, perfectionistic, and stern. Ms. DD loved to play the violin, and her parents vigorously encouraged her talent. Their pleasure in her growing artistry seemed to soften the strained and harsh atmosphere within the family for a time. Further, Ms. DD became quite attached to her violin teacher, who seemed a warmer, livelier presence than either of her parents. However, she soon found that her pleasure in her artistry began to recede as her parents and even her teacher seemed increasingly focused on her technical performance, her hours practicing, and an increasingly demanding schedule of public performances showcasing her abilities.

Ms. DD also felt confused about the impact of her abilities on others. Peers seemed envious or resentful when she was praised by her teachers, and Ms. DD felt torn between an aggressive desire to be admired for her talents and a wish to simply disappear from the limelight in order to "fit in."

In late adolescence, Ms. DD abandoned her nascent musical career. She felt guilty about this decision, because it seemed to greatly disappoint her parents and violin teacher. She also felt somewhat adrift. Shortly after she left for college, Ms. DD began to feel depressed.

Her treatment, initiated some years later when she was 31, focused on an exploration of her perfectionism:

> Ms. DD: I think I really do see things in black and white. If I'm not out there anymore, winning awards for the violin, I think that no one will ever notice me. I feel like an invisible nobody. I guess that's because I felt for so long that it was the only thing that really mattered to my parents and to my teacher, even though I realize that's not really true. Now, I seem to feel as if I have only those two choices: to be perfect in every way and to please everyone, like I did with my music, or to be nobody and feel bad about myself. And since I'm not even playing anymore, I'm not sure I ever *could* get back to where I was. I feel there is nothing special or successful about me now. That's scary.

Ms. DD's treatment focused first on her perfectionism, because her depression seemed to intensify every time she perceived herself as failing to conform to excruciatingly high standards of commendable behavior. These standards concerned not only moral behavior but also almost every aspect of her dress, her comportment, and her capabilities. Her perceived failures were accompanied by guilt but particularly by a pervasive sense of shame.

Therapist and patient became quickly aware that Ms. DD's perfectionism reflected a strong wish to win others' approval and support and to deflect their anger. Idealization can often play a role in attempting to manage conflicted anger, either to modulate anger at others or others toward the self. This was easily connected to Ms. DD's considerable fear of her father's disapproval and physical punishments, as well as to her attempts to maintain a connection with her depressed and distracted mother and with the idealized violin teacher. Ms. DD easily recognized some of the compensatory aspects of her perfectionism but still felt trapped by this dynamic:

> Ms. DD: I spent so much time trying to please my parents, to get their attention through my music, that I didn't really know how to connect with other kids. I think I tried to compensate for that by drawing attention to myself in terms of my violin. Like, "Look what I can do!" or "Who needs *you* when

I'm so special?" I just can't continue with all that: it feels so
self-centered. But now what? If I'm not perfect and I'm not
winning awards, my parents get upset and I feel that no one
else really likes me anyway.... It feels like there's no way out
of this trap.

Working to understand the less obvious dynamics connected with her
perfectionism was quite helpful for Ms. DD. She gradually revealed a long-
standing sense of emptiness, frustrated anger, and helplessness in the face
of her parents' chronic discord and personal unhappiness. Her pleasure in
a soaring musical talent had seemed to reassure Ms. DD that she was neither empty nor lacking in femininity herself, as she had sadly perceived her
rather depressed mother to be. Her musical interests also provided her a
warmer, more responsive woman with whom to identify, in her violin teacher,
although this connection did seem contingent, to a degree, on her native
talent. Further, the beauty of her music seemed to counteract what Ms. DD
perceived to be the harshness of her frustration and anger with her parents,
particularly with her punitive father.

However, when parents and teacher began to insist on increasing standards of perfection in her performance, Ms. DD felt deeply disappointed,
even at times humiliated, as her talents no longer seemed to ensure the
approving connection and sense of power they once afforded. She became
resentful, and her anger began to contaminate what had been previously
a source of pure pride and pleasure.

Further, when pursuing her musical career began to demand more competitive aggression, Ms. DD experienced this aggression as harsh, grasping,
and unfeminine. She was dimly aware of growing fantasies about acclaim
and vindication, of becoming more powerful than her aggressive father, her
unhappy mother, or her unresponsive peers. The aggression in these fantasies increasingly interfered with the pleasure, harmony, and self-respect that
pursuing music had once afforded her. Without the power and affirmation
her talents brought, however, Ms. DD felt powerless, essentially castrated,
and therefore degraded.

In therapy, Ms. DD gradually learned to differentiate a healthy competitiveness from the deep, reactive rage she had felt toward her parents,
teacher, and peers. This enabled her to become more comfortable with self-
assertion in many realms. Ms. DD also began to recognize how much she
had invested in her musical talent as her only potential source of power and
femininity and how she consequently viewed herself as devalued when
there was no ongoing proof of the extent of her abilities. Understanding the
context of her need to idealize or devalue enabled Ms. DD to relax her perfectionism to a considerable extent, although she continued to work on

this, even after her successful treatment. As noted in the studies of Blatt et al. (2010) (see Chapter 12, "Psychodynamic Approaches to Depression With Comorbid Personality Disorder"), perfectionism can be a persistent problem and may require longer-term treatment to address.

Case Example 2

Ms. EE was a single, middle-aged caterer who had been involved in a frustrating relationship with a lawyer, Larry, for several years. She had imagined that on her fortieth birthday, he would propose to her, despite the knowledge that this was highly unlikely. Larry had made it all too clear that to the contrary, he thought of marriage as an ensnaring catastrophe. His own parents had been desperately unhappy together: Long periods of mutual bitterness punctuated by physical battles had made his family life intolerable.

As her birthday approached, Ms. EE became increasingly depressed as she realized that her fantasy would never materialize. She gradually replaced that idea with another: If Larry would not marry her, at least he could buy her the dress of her dreams—a beautiful designer gown that they had looked at together while on vacation. Larry had the means to provide this, and Ms. EE decided that this would be the only acceptable compensation for her forbearance.

Her therapist explored the meaning of these fantasies with her patient.

MS. EE: Marriage…you know, my parents weren't very happy together, either. And I don't know that I'm desperate to have children, except that I really don't want to be alone in my old age. But…all my friends are married, and I feel like an outsider. Like nothing. It's embarrassing. I keep imagining that dress…it's so perfect. I guess I understand that Larry will never agree to marriage. And it's not like he would be so easy to live with. But I have given up a lot for him, and I deserve something! He knows how much I want that gown. I feel as if people would look at me differently if he gave me that. I would feel…proud. And if I can't have a wedding dress, at least I can wear that gown when we go to dances at his firm.

THERAPIST: It sounds as if you are looking for proof that you can show others that you are valued—as if without that beautiful dress, you are nothing.

MS. EE: I do feel like that. If my appearance isn't perfect or my clothes aren't beautiful, I think that people will look down on me. Anytime I get a bad haircut, I cringe and I really don't even want to leave the house.

Her therapist worked hard with Ms. EE over many years on this aspect of her dynamics, which was deeply entrenched. This patient had also grown up in a parental battlefield, in which her embittered mother frequently accused her father of failing to provide adequately for the family. His failure to buy the family a house had come to represent, in a very concrete way, other, more subtle failures within the family in achieving warmth and emotional connection.

Ms. EE often felt overlooked and alone as her parents were battling and seemed to have felt chronically empty, deprived of a nourishing, individual attention. Now, she searched for material evidence that she was valued and seen as special. Interpretations of her rage and consequent guilt were much easier for Ms. EE to understand and accept than interpretations about her fantasies concerning value and perfection. This pattern can occur in patients with perfectionism and idealization, as they might not recognize a tendency that has been active subconsciously over many years. Ms. EE persisted in believing that she needed to demonstrate her value to the world through her connection with the idealized boyfriend's wealth and power, through "perfect" gifts or through attributes of physical beauty. Without these, she felt certain that she was a denigrated failure, a "loser" in the eyes of the world. As Ms. EE became older and some of her attributes of beauty began to fade, her susceptibility to depression increased.

Rothstein (1984) notes that "sicker" patients with narcissistic personality disorder are often "devoid of an ego ideal in the traditional sense of the word...[but] remain fixated on concrete self-...representations" (p. 57). In other words, rather than holding themselves to an evolving set of standards or principles, such patients often remain focused on achieving rather concrete goals, such as attaining wealth or fame or beauty, in order to feel valuable or valued. Helping patients recognize the limitations in such aspirations is extremely difficult, although it is still well worth attempting to bring these dynamics to the patient's attention. Even though Ms. EE continued to hold rather rigidly to concrete images of material or physical perfection that she imagined would confer value, she did feel somewhat helped by recognizing this dynamic. For instance, she relinquished some of her material demands on her boyfriend, relieving considerable pressure on their relationship.

Addressing Idealization and Devaluation of Others

In focused psychotherapy for depression, it is important to help patients identify tendencies to idealize or devalue selected others. Exploring this tendency often reveals that it is a strategy for ignoring painful feelings about loved ones or about the patients themselves or for bolstering low self-esteem. The resulting distortion in their perceptions of interpersonal reality may leave depressed patients confused, disappointed, and vulnerable. Further, cycles of idealization and disappointment may burden their relationships and cause others to distance themselves, intensifying a sense of rejection or guilt.

Case Example 3

Dr. FF was a successful young physician in his early 30s. A year before starting treatment, he had married Cara, a beautiful woman who worked in his field. Dr. FF had been "swept off his feet" by her and noted particularly how much he loved and admired her family, who were vibrant, successful, and very close. Dr. FF contrasted them with his family; his parents had divorced. His mother had left his father in a rage about the man's failings, and Dr. FF concurred that in fact, his father was a deeply flawed man. The entire family struggled financially, and Dr. FF's siblings, whom he tended to avoid, now lived constricted and embittered lives. Dr. FF was delighted, in contrast, by Cara's family, with whom he spent increasing amounts of time during the couple's engagement.

After the two married, however, Dr. FF began to feel upset about the demands of inclusion in his new family. An outgoing and close-knit group, they tended to spend every weekend together, playing sports, dining, and talking late into the night. Dr. FF, who had at first been exhilarated by this, began to fear that he would never be able to keep up. He was often tired from the demands of his work and enjoyed downtime, during which he could read or take long, solitary walks. He began to fear that he was "odd and bookish" and would not fit in with this idealized group. Further, he craved separate, intimate time with his wife, who seemed to prefer the company of her ebullient family to quiet afternoons with him. In this context, Dr. FF became progressively more depressed, torn between devaluing himself and devaluing the family he once idealized. At times, he lashed out in angry criticisms toward his wife, calling her "shallow and unsupportive," but later would feel agonized, guilty, and even more demeaned in his own view.

> DR. FF: I feel like such a disappointment to my wife and her family. I wanted so much to be like them; they are just perfect together. Instead, I feel like a complete failure. When Cara complains about my anger or about my need for downtime, it makes me feel as if she thinks I'm a stick-in-the-mud or an angry malcontent.
>
> THERAPIST: I'm sure it brings up, in your mind, your mother's accusations of your father—that he was asocial and difficult.

DR. FF: I never wanted to be like that! Maybe I'm doomed to be like him. This feels awful.

The therapist then took note of her patient's tendency to idealize others and their style of conducting their lives, leading to shameful feelings about himself for being different. She also noted the alternation of such assessments with a tendency to devalue these same others when they disappointed him.

THERAPIST: When you think about how much you want to be like your wife and her family, your desire to have some periods of solitude, to read, or to be alone with your wife seems *shameful*. When you're angry, I suspect you feel differently. I think you are not convinced, deep down, that those pursuits are necessarily so bad. When you're angry with your wife, I think you are disappointed and hurt that she doesn't want to spend more time with you or that she doesn't appreciate your quiet side. Then, you start to devalue *her* in your mind. *She* becomes the big disappointment, and it's hard to keep in mind her appealing qualities.

DR. FF: It's true. I do feel that way at those times, and I just erupt and attack her. But later, I feel so terrible about it! She's not a bad or shallow person at all. It's *me*. *I* feel like the angry misanthrope.

THERAPIST: It sounds as if, in your view, things get pretty polarized. Either your wife and her family are perfect, ideal people and you are a loser, or you're entirely right and *she* is the disappointment.

DR. FF: When you say it like that, it sounds like everything is too black and white for me. I always thought that was a strength. I love my mom, but she can't find the fault in anyone, other than maybe my father, and is always getting dumped on. I like to be discriminating. I like to have standards.

The therapist then tried to link Dr. FF's "black and white" assessments of others with some of his underlying fears and noted how unrealistic his standards could be and how threatening deviations from these standards could become.[1]

THERAPIST: So, you want to be different from your father, who disappointed you by being aloof and cranky. And you want

---

[1] The dynamics include Jacobson's (1971) (see Chapter 2) conception that depressed patients can be highly self-critical of any aspects of their attitudes or behavior that they see as linked to those they despised in their parents.

to be different from your mother, who lets people take advantage of her. If you detect *anything* resembling those qualities in yourself, you're concerned that you'll be deserted, as your dad was, or taken advantage of, like your mother. Your only way out is to be really special: a highly successful physician; a model son-in-law and husband. But if you are not completely—one hundred percent—up to these standards, then you feel like a horrible failure! I agree with you that standards are important, but I think that if you or others don't completely measure up to your standards, it feels very bad, very threatening to you, far out of proportion to what is actually occurring.

In this vignette, intertwining dynamics are demonstrated. The first concerns Dr. FF's perfectionism. At this point, early in his treatment, there were preliminary indications about vulnerabilities and fantasies linked to his compensatory need for marked success and for affiliation with idealized, successful others. From the limited history available, it seemed that Dr. FF needed to avoid the sense of failure and abandonment connected with his father and the sense of humiliation or passivity that he connected with attributes of his mother. Dr. FF *did* seem propelled to accumulate evidence that he was a highly valued citizen, professional, husband, and son-in-law and, in the absence of this evidence, to feel degraded and ashamed. Similarly, when disappointed by his idealized new family, Dr. FF tended to experience a frustrated rage and to see his wife in a devalued way. This caused her to distance herself from him, exacerbating his depression.

As long as Dr. FF held rigidly polarized visions of himself and others, accessing more complex fantasies about himself and his parents was quite difficult. Considerable work had to be done first to help him understand the limitations of his ideas of value and idealized perfection and to see the connection of these viewpoints to his troubles with his wife and to his depression.

Case Example 4

Mr. GG, 35 years old, was part of a talented family, with several members who were well known in their fields of academic endeavor. His peers in academia were well aware of the family's prominence, and Mr. GG both enjoyed this knowledge and felt burdened by it. When he published a book in the shared area and received some acclaim, he was delighted but frightened about having to live up to "exalted expectations" of himself in the future.

Mr. GG was also burdened by the meanings his success seemed to hold for his mother. He suspected that he had always been favored among his siblings, and now his mother seemed to acknowledge this openly. She seemed excessively preoccupied with his success, as if it were her own. Again, Mr. GG felt delighted but also angry, frightened, and confused. Particularly difficult for him was the fact that he was receiving much more acclaim than had his father, whose reputation in his department had been secure because of his many books and articles, but who never had published a book that received the attention outside of academia that his son's had.

Mr. GG had been engaged in a long-term relationship with a loving woman, but with his success, she began to diminish in his eyes. He wondered openly whether she would prove to be "enough" for him, and began to "secretly" date other women. Once she learned of this, his girlfriend ended their relationship, expressing shock, hurt, and anger.[2]

Mr. GG became depressed and was referred for treatment. In his initial interview, he described his depression as originating from the breakup with his girlfriend.

> THERAPIST: I agree that your depression has a lot to do with what happened with you and your girlfriend. Can you tell me more about that?
>
> MR. GG: I feel like a shit. She was terrific, and I really hurt her. I can imagine that you think I'm this awful, predatory man. That's what her friends think. But I just couldn't commit to her, once I started thinking that at some point she wouldn't be enough for me. I started to see her differently. I couldn't feel attracted to her anymore. It all felt like a lie. It felt awful.
>
> THERAPIST: How *did* you begin to see her?
>
> MR. GG: She started to seem boring, not very lively. I really need someone who's quick, who thinks as fast as I do, and who's very responsive to help me feel alive. I was feeling held back.
>
> THERAPIST: Can you tell me more about *that* feeling? Is that familiar?
>
> MR. GG: Yes, I feel it all the time. Restless. I like it when someone gets my sense of humor and can keep up with it.
>
> THERAPIST: And if they don't?
>
> MR. GG: Things feel flat, dead. I hate that feeling.
>
> THERAPIST: It sounds as if that's a very familiar feeling. Does it go way back?

---

[2]Although Mr. GG's attitude may be a trait of narcissistic personality disorder ("Believes that he or she is 'special' and unique and can only be understood by, or should associate with, other special or high-status people [or institutions]" in DSM-5 [American Psychiatric Association 2013]), the therapist employing this treatment would work to identify underlying factors contributing to the dynamics of the overlapping symptoms and character traits (see Chapter 12).

MR. GG: Yes! I guess I felt it a lot when I was alone. My parents used to go off on a lot of trips and to leave me with a babysitter. I hated that nanny! Anyway, they'd go off and I would be pathetic—howling, crying. My mother couldn't deal with it, and I felt stupid. And that babysitter would get angry and send me alone to my room. I felt bad, flat....When I was older, I'd get angry and break things.

In this vignette, exploring Mr. GG's current disenchantment with his girlfriend led to information about the loneliness, rage, and sadness that had accompanied his frequent early separations from his parents. Mr. GG felt helpless, small, and ashamed of his needy reactions, which had been viewed with distaste by all around him. His parents' absence had left a dreaded "flat" feeling that he struggled to avoid by all means possible. As he grew older, Mr. GG sought to surround himself with engaging people whose presence was enlivening in order to ward off the reappearance of such empty, deadening feelings. Until recently, he had often considered his girlfriend to be such a person.

THERAPIST: I wonder why your view of her changed *now*. It seems to have something to do with your success.

MR. GG: Well, sure. I feel like now, at the college, people *look* at me. It's not just that they are noticing my family; it's *me*. Soon enough, I'll start getting the other end of it, people expecting a home run every time I publish a book and getting disappointed! When I think about all that, I'm just not sure about Linda. I want someone who I will always feel proud to be with.

THERAPIST: The idea of feeling proud and of wanting Linda to be "up to it" seems to come up when you imagine people *looking* at you, with admiration or with criticism, then?

MR. GG: Yes.

THERAPIST: Maybe you want to be sure that you will be with someone who *never* feels like *you* felt when your parents were away and you felt so small and helpless and alone. If *she* is powerful and can never feel humiliated, maybe then you won't ever feel that way, either. Then, when people look at you, they will see someone solid and important.

Other dynamics contributed to Mr. GG's breakup, apart from his powerful need to idealize or devalue others as he himself felt idealized or degraded. His therapist suspected that Mr. GG felt guilty about his competitive victory over siblings and father and uncomfortable with his mother's undisguised favoritism. She thought that this guilt, plus ambivalent feelings toward women stimulated by Mr. GG's confusing relationship with his mother, also led him to devalue Linda. These feelings and the fantasies connected with them were also explored within this treatment. However, identifying the tendency to idealize or devalue others remained a primary focus for the duration of Mr. GG's treatment.

Exploring Idealization and Devaluation in the Transference

As with other dynamic constellations, the transference is an important area for exploring idealization and devaluation.

Case Example 5

Ms. HH was a married novelist in her 30s with three small children when she presented with significant depression and marital conflict.

The oldest of three, Ms. HH had been extremely close to her alcoholic mother. This woman, it seemed, was attractive, lively, dramatic, and self-absorbed, with behavior that ranged from delightful to maddening. Her erratic enthusiasms dominated household conversation and included an obsession with religious mysticism and the theater. Ms. HH often felt excited about her mother's sweeping enthusiasms and recalled her mother's habit of awakening her at midnight, even on school nights, to keep her company watching television until the early morning hours.

During her adolescence, Ms. HH repudiated her mother with a vengeance, then seeing her enthusiasms as embarrassing and becoming painfully aware of her alcoholic symptoms, which included vindictive outbursts alternating with solipsistic reveries and passing out in the living room in the early evenings. Ms. HH turned her attention toward her father, an apparently vain and somewhat paranoid man who seemed largely uninvolved with their family life, except for delivering occasional withering criticisms of his children's behavior. Her attempts to engage him were at times briefly satisfying but often frustrating or confusing. His teasing or admiring comments about her developing body, for instance, were both exciting and scary to Ms. HH, and she vacillated between inviting or retreating from them.

In Ms. HH's current life, marital difficulties and a relentless perfectionism about her writing contributed to a chronic sense of misery. She idealized her husband, a lawyer, as powerful and brilliant, but Ms. HH found his lack of sexual desire infuriating: the couple rarely made love. She became involved in an affair with another novelist, whom she found sexy but untalented. Ms. HH was conflicted and guilty about her affair, but even more guilty about her con-

tempt for what she saw as her husband's sexual passivity and her lover's immaturity and lack of genuine talent. Finally, Ms. HH alternated between
moments of great intimacy and a sense of hostile, beleaguered distance from
her children, significantly frustrating them and paining her husband.

Ms. HH came to understand in therapy her tendency to both idealize
and devalue the important figures in her life as linked to her intense disappointment and rage toward both parents. Ms. HH had experienced little
middle ground between admiring her bewitching and vibrant mother or de-
spising her for her weaknesses, revealed only too clearly when she was drunk.
Her father had offered his daughter little emotional support, but she had
vainly attempted to discover in him at least a model for identification. However, her sadness, anxiety, and confusion about his criticism and intrusive
sexual comments caused her to retreat, and she now found it difficult to see
or understand him without a defensive veneer of contempt.

As Ms. HH slowly realized that her contempt disguised more complex feelings of need, admiration, anger, and perplexed but profound disappointment,
she was able to gradually view her parents and others in her life in a more realistic way. She relinquished her affair and entered marital treatment with her
husband to explore ways of communicating about her disappointment in their
sexual relationship and about her difficulties with their children.

However, Ms. HH's relentless devaluation of her writing continued to
make her working life a misery. Attempts to explore the states of deflation
and emptiness that plagued her as she assessed her work were met with intense resistance. Similarly, Ms. HH could only intellectually acknowledge
feelings of vulnerability and helplessness experienced in the face of her parents' self-absorption.

> MS. HH: I know you think I felt sad about my parents' lack of at-
> tention. But really I don't remember ever actually feeling
> that way. When I think about staying up late at night with
> my mother, it feels like it was *fun*. I just can't connect at all
> to the fact that it was selfish of her—that I probably was
> tired and couldn't focus in school the next day.

Similarly, although Ms. HH seemed to feel attached to her therapist,
she struggled to negate this feeling and seemed to oscillate, almost moment to moment at times, between idealizing and denigrating her.

> MS. HH: I think that you're really helpful, and I do feel like you're
> always there. But there's something about that that I also
> find disgusting. Too feminine. Weak.
> THERAPIST: I know that if you acted as though you needed some-
> thing in your family, you often became the butt of jokes.
> You've mentioned that when you asked for the same thing
> for your birthday several years in a row, your parents joked

that they would keep forgetting to get it for you. It must have seemed foolish to want anything too much. So, if *I want* to look with you at how that felt, I *also* seem foolish and weak.

MS. HH: I guess so. I really don't want to talk about this. It's like my parents all over again. You want to talk about *you*. There's no way for this to be helpful.

Ms. HH resisted efforts to explore these feelings further and began to consider termination, pointing out that she was doing much better in her marriage and felt generally less depressed, alienated, and contemptuous. Her therapist thought that Ms. HH, though improved, remained at risk for a depressive relapse, because she still had times of great emptiness and self-condemnation. During the period in which they had been discussing termination, Ms. HH called in crisis one Saturday morning.

MS. HH: I've been drinking and I didn't want to tell you about it. In the evenings, I've been drinking about a half bottle of wine. Last night, I think I blacked out. It feels like I'm becoming my mother.

During their next sessions, her therapist persisted in exploring the transferential meanings of Ms. HH's secretive drinking.

THERAPIST: Can you tell me how it felt, keeping this a secret?

MS. HH: I think it was exciting, like I was "getting over on you." You can't be too helpful if you can't even figure out that I'm drinking. But I know that you aren't a mind reader.... You can't figure it out unless I tell you.

THERAPIST: I think that you are stuck going back and forth between the idea that *someone* in a relationship must be powerful and exciting, and someone else, weak, empty, helpless. It's either you who are the *powerful* one, like your mother felt to you sometimes—so exciting, so alive, knowing so much about so many secret, adult things—and I am helpless, foolish, left out, not knowing which end is up. Or I must be a powerful mind reader [from whom] you are waiting for help when you feel so empty and bad. When I don't read your mind in some magical way, I'm a big disappointment, and you're really upset and furious with me.

MS. HH: Yes. And I can show everyone how stupid you are by telling them that you never picked up on my drinking. My husband thinks you must not know what you're doing.

Many dimensions of Ms. HH's narcissism were enacted in this episode. She felt terrified of her needy and helpless feelings and projected them onto her therapist, instead of allowing herself to experience them. Thus, Ms. HH felt that her therapist was the needy loser, who needed and wanted her to feel unacceptable things rather than simply, magically making her feel whole. Ms. HH longed for her therapist to reveal herself as the omnipotent, caring mother about whom she had fantasized in childhood and was enraged when this did not occur.

This transference dynamic needed to be explored again and again in Ms. HH's treatment, from multiple vantage points. The exploration seemed to be quite helpful in many respects, because Ms. HH improved considerably during the course of a lengthy psychotherapy in terms of her marital relationship, her relationship with her children, and even her work. However, there was a repetitive quality to the transference enactments, as if Ms. HH could not bear to give up her search for an idealized parent, nor her rage about the attendant frustration. Indeed, she ended her treatment in the middle of an angry interaction with her therapist over an increase in her fees, although she did later call to apologize and was able to reflect on her anger. Her therapist felt concerned about this ending to the treatment but did think, nonetheless, that many of the insights gained through the transference work had been helpful to Ms. HH, and she hoped that Ms. HH would be able to continue to make use of them in her life or in her work with a different therapist.

References

American Psychiatric Association: Diagnostic and Statistical Manual of Mental Disorders, 5th Edition. Arlington, VA, American Psychiatric Association, 2013

Arieti S, Bemporad J: Severe and Mild Depression: The Psychotherapeutic Approach. New York, Basic Books, 1978

Blatt SJ, Zuroff DC, Hawley LL, Auerbach JS: Predictors of sustained therapeutic change. Psychother Res 20(1):37–54, 2010 19757328

Jacobson E: Depression: Comparative Studies of Normal, Neurotic, and Psychotic Conditions. New York, International Universities Press, 1971

Kohut H: The Analysis of the Self. New York, International Universities Press, 1971

Milrod D: The wished-for self image. Psychoanal Study Child 37:95–120, 1982 7178328

Reich A: Pathologic forms of self-esteem regulation. Psychoanal Study Child 15:215–232, 1960 13740410

Rothstein A: The Narcissistic Pursuit of Perfection, 2nd Edition, Revised. New York, International Universities Press, 1984

10

Defense Mechanisms in Depressed Patients

AS discussed in Chapter 2 ("Development of a Psychodynamic Model of Depression"), patients prone to depression use a number of defense mechanisms that can be usefully recognized for therapeutic work as habitual ways of protecting themselves from conscious comprehension of warded-off affects and fantasies (Bloch et al. 1993). Although these defenses may temporarily ease painful feelings, in the long term they can worsen depressive symptoms. As described in Chapter 9 ("Idealization and Devaluation"), for example, idealization employed in an effort to bolster self-esteem or protect others from aggression may lead to disappointment and devaluation when self and others cannot meet the inflated expectations. Therefore, it is important to help patients become aware of characteristic defenses and more directly access underlying, threatening fantasies. As long as patients avoid awareness of their anger, for example, it is difficult to help them view anger as less toxic or to help them keep from turning the anger against themselves. Defense mechanisms employed by depressed patients typically include denial, projection, idealization and devaluation, passive aggression, identification with the aggressor, and reaction formation (Table 10–1) (Bloch et al. 1993; Brenner 1975; Jacobson 1971). Idealization and devaluation are discussed separately in Chapter 9.

Table 10–1. Defense mechanisms in depression

Denial	Anger or other strong feelings or perceptions are not recognized, interfering with their effective acknowledgment and expression.
Projection	Thoughts and feelings are denied and experienced as coming from others. When angry feelings are projected, this may intensify depression as others are experienced as rejecting.
Passive aggression	Anger is expressed indirectly via withholding behaviors, including procrastination.
Identification with the aggressor	Identification with someone experienced as powerful and aggressive often triggers guilty reactions.
Reaction formation	Feelings such as anger are denied and converted into their opposite—for example, a positive helpfulness. However, the anger can then become self-directed.

Denial

Denial is a core defense mechanism of depressed patients, employed particularly as a means of avoiding hostile and destructive feelings or fantasies. This mechanism is used primarily to keep the experience of anger from consciousness. Patients may also attempt to deny feelings of low self-esteem or narcissistic vulnerability, however, even as they appear to struggle with these feelings intensely. As described in the first case example below, patients' denial of anger usually does not effectively avert depression, as the inability to experience anger toward others is associated with its deflection toward the self. In addition, patients cannot adequately address their concerns or frustrations with others, which frequently interferes with the negotiation of needs in interpersonal relationships and ultimately contributes to feelings of ineffectiveness and poor self-esteem. Therapists should explore denied feelings with patients and help them more effectively tolerate and manage their anger.

Case Example 1

Ms. II, a 32-year-old sales agent, had recurrent major depressive episodes over many years. Although she felt frustrated with the men she dated and with problems at her job, Ms. II was not very aware of these feelings and tended to behave passive aggressively (see below) by, for example, being quite late or canceling appointments with others. Her friends and coworkers in turn became frustrated with Ms. II and distanced themselves from her emotionally. She would then feel treated unfairly, escalating her sense of inadequacy.

Ms. II's depression had intensified with the death of her mother about 5 years earlier. Ms. II denied any anger at her mother and spoke of missing her terribly since her death, particularly her mother's support in dealing with the problems in her life. Nevertheless, as exploration proceeded, significant negative feelings about her mother emerged. Ms. II recalled being treated at times like the black sheep of the family, because her mother would sometimes criticize her for apparently little reason. For example, she once explosively attacked Ms. II for failing to do the laundry when the patient felt that she had not been assigned this chore. In another instance, her mother castigated her for keeping a messy room, comparing her negatively with her siblings.

Ms. II began to realize that she was quite angry with her mother and found this frightening and guilt provoking. How could she feel so angry at someone to whom she also felt so close and who was no longer around to defend herself? In this context, Ms. II reported a very vivid and powerfully affecting dream:

Ms. II: I am going on a train with my mother. She begins to criticize me for not having gotten the right tickets. I start screaming at her in a very loud manner, and she backs off. Pretty soon I'm screaming at everyone: the conductor, other passengers, and my father, who has appeared in the dream.

THERAPIST: What feelings do you have about this dream?

Ms. II: Well, I'd expect I'd feel terrible, but in fact, I felt really relieved. I've never been able to yell at anyone like that. And I'm beginning to feel that my mother does deserve some of this. I'm starting to recall more episodes of her picking on me needlessly.

THERAPIST: It seems as if one concern that you've had is that if you get angry at all, it would come out in a way that felt completely out of control.

Ms. II: That's true. But here I am doing it in the dream, and I don't really feel bad about it. Plus, I think maybe I can control this anger better.

THERAPIST: It also seems that if you bring up your frustrations with people as they occur, your anger wouldn't build up so much.

This dream represented an important breakthrough for Ms. II in the lifting of her denial of long-standing rageful feelings. As is usually the case with patients, this important insight did not lead to an immediate change in her behavior. It did, however, provide a valuable framework as Ms. II became increasingly able to address her frustrations with others and to understand her fears of damage and attack and her guilt that were associated with these assertions.

Projection

In employing projection, patients deny specific feelings and fantasies and instead perceive them as coming from external forces or from others within their environment. Depressed patients typically project their anger onto others. This may help them feel safer and less guilty with regard to their own aggression but nonetheless leads them to experience their world as hostile and rejecting. In a vicious cycle, the sense of hostility and rejection from others intensifies patients' anger and leads to further projection of an even more hostile external environment, escalating a sense of helplessness and depression. In addressing this defense, the therapist helps patients understand how these hostile feelings and fantasies originate within themselves, allowing for more effective management of these feelings.

Case Example 2

Ms. C, discussed in Chapters 2 ("Development of a Psychodynamic Model of Depression") and 3 ("Overview of Psychodynamic Psychotherapy for Depression"), regularly saw others in her environment as hostile toward her. She viewed herself as a victim of unfair treatment by others and denied feeling angry at them, experiencing herself instead as being suddenly attacked without provocation. A vivid example occurred at her job, where she experienced her boss as tormenting her. However, it steadily emerged in her treatment that Ms. C was engaged in a veritable sit-down strike there, often coming in late and showing little enthusiasm for the work she was given. She would even covertly defy some of the rules that her boss set, such as taking extra long coffee breaks.

> THERAPIST: Don't you think these things would make your boss angry?
>
> MS. C: Well, I don't see why they should. I get my work done. It's still not fair that she's always attacking me. Besides, she criticizes me about every little thing, not just what you're describing. And most of the criticisms don't make sense.
>
> THERAPIST: I wonder if your defying her in some areas may trigger her anger toward you more generally.
>
> MS. C: Well, it wouldn't be fair, then, just to attack me about things that aren't really a problem.
>
> THERAPIST: It does sound as if you're angry at her.
>
> MS. C: Well, maybe. Mostly I just feel hurt. I don't get where this is coming from.

As can be seen, the patient significantly denied her anger and viewed the hostility as operating in one direction only: from her boss toward her. Ms. C's denial and the projection of her anger made it difficult for her to recognize that her feelings and behaviors might be provoking her boss's wrath.

The therapist was able to make some progress with Ms. C as he explored her rebellious behaviors further. Ms. C described how she and her colleagues would get together and make fun of their boss.

THERAPIST: What do you say about her?

MS. C: Well, we talk about how stupid and arrogant she is. She had me read something she wrote. I thought it was useless, and I guess she felt it was really important. At our meeting, she asked me to discuss what value I found in it. I said I didn't see any.

THERAPIST: How did she respond?

MS. C: She seemed very upset. Later in the conversation, she suggested I look for a job in another department.

THERAPIST: From what you're describing, it would be hard for you to claim you're not angry at her.

MS. C: Well, I guess so. Since we talked about it, I've really felt the angry feelings.

THERAPIST: My sense is you also want to make her feel bad. You want to hurt her, just as you feel she is hurtful to you.

MS. C: Do you think so? I don't like to think of myself in that way.

THERAPIST: In what way?

MS. C: As an angry, hurtful person.

THERAPIST: Perhaps then you feel you are too much like your mother.

MS. C: Maybe. That's an awful thought for me. She was always attacking and alienating others.

For this patient, recognizing her hostility was painful but also quite valuable. It helped Ms. C to stop provoking her boss and to recognize the threat that her poorly managed anger presented for her. Gradually, she learned more effective means of coping with her discontent and frustration. Ms. C also began to realize that the retaliation that she provoked from others served as a punishment for her angry feelings, about which she felt extremely guilty and ashamed because of their link to her mother's damaging aggression. Ms. C struggled in this regard with an identification with the aggressor, a mechanism that is described further below.

Passive Aggression

Another means by which patients can defend against conflicted aggression is the mechanism of passive aggression. Patients express their anger indirectly through passively provocative behaviors, allowing them to deny how intensely angry they actually feel. Ms. II's and Ms. C's tardiness at work are examples of passive-aggressive behaviors. This mechanism is intended to reduce patients' imagined risk from more overt displays of aggression. It serves, too, to deny anger or to enact it in ways that patients consider less hurtful. As with other mechanisms used in depression, however, it tends to backfire. Patients do not experience the relief that a more effective expression of grievances would provide, and others are often provoked by their passivity, increasing the patients' experience of interpersonal difficulties against which they feel helpless.

Case Example 3

Mr. JJ, a 56-year-old married accountant with dysthymia, was greatly frustrated with his wife. He felt that she had not responded to him sexually early in their marriage and that she continued to regard him without passion or deep love. Mr. JJ seemed on a long-standing quest to retaliate against his wife by withholding sex and by not taking care of himself or performing professionally as she hoped he would. The patient had difficulty admitting that these behaviors were intended as revenge.

> MR. JJ: When we went into the marriage, I wanted to have sex with her, and she wasn't responsive to me. So why would I want to respond to her needs now?
>
> THERAPIST: It sounds as if you're trying to get back at her.
>
> MR. JJ: Well, I guess I am, in a way. I don't usually think of it like that. I really think of myself as a nice guy.
>
> THERAPIST: Does she know about your frustrations with her?
>
> MR. JJ: Not really. I mean, she's frustrated about my not responding to her sexually, but I haven't really told her why. I mean, what you're calling the revenge thing.
>
> THERAPIST: Why not?
>
> MR. JJ: I don't really want to hurt her feelings. I think it would make her feel really bad.
>
> THERAPIST: But it sounds like that's the net effect of your withholding sexually anyway.
>
> MR. JJ: Yes. I guess so.

Through these clarifications, Mr. JJ was ultimately able to see that his behavior toward his wife was vengeful, even though he expressed it in a passive, withholding manner. A major problem with Mr. JJ's approach was that he furthered his own feelings of inadequacy by not dealing more effectively and directly with his wife. In fact, he blocked his own professional success, further alienating his wife, and received even less support from her than he might have otherwise.

Identification With the Aggressor

In employing the defense mechanism of identifying with an aggressor, patients connect their own image of themselves with that of an aggressive individual, particularly someone who has had power over them in the past. Patients who feel vulnerable or inadequate may identify with an aggressor in an attempt to gain a sense of adequacy and control. However, guilty feelings are often triggered by such an identification. The following case illustrates the latter phenomenon.

Case Example 4

Mr. W, a lawyer with dysthymia who is discussed in Chapter 7, "Addressing Angry Reactions to Narcissistic Injury" (see Case Example 4), had significant difficulty getting his staff members to complete their tasks properly. He wanted to be seen as a friend rather than a boss. He accepted weak excuses for their need to leave early or take days off and was very accepting of shoddy work. However, he would tend to obsess angrily about his employees' not adequately doing their job and blamed them in part for the limited success of his practice. Occasionally he would mildly reproach one of them.

> THERAPIST: Why do you think you have difficulty making more demands on your employees?
> MR. W: Well, I'm scared they'll quit and then I'll be stuck training a new person. I also want to be seen as the good guy. I don't want to hurt their feelings.
> THERAPIST: What do you mean by that?
> MR. W: I feel like if I criticize them, I'll get really nasty or abusive and just make them feel very badly.
> THERAPIST: I think it's important for us to understand more about this.

Mr. W's background, discussed in more depth in Chapter 7, again proved relevant to this issue. He described his parents as very unfair and rigid about rules. He was often upbraided about minor infractions (coming home a few minutes late for curfew) or for not making better grades, even though he found school difficult. He was furious with his parents, but if he got angry directly, his mother would "withdraw her love" and not speak to him for days. This caused him great anguish, and he struggled between his wish to be a "good boy" and his anger at what he regarded as unfair treatment. The therapist discussed with Mr. W how viewing himself as an assertive boss was identified in his mind with his parents' criticisms of him.

> THERAPIST: It's interesting that when you describe yourself as a boss critiquing your employees, your behavior sounds just like your parents' with you.
>
> MR. W: Yes. I guess it does. I mean, I don't want to be unfair and to hurt people the way they did with me. I know what it feels like.
>
> THERAPIST: It sounds as if you really feel guilty when you need to critique your employees, even though you actually tend to be overly polite.
>
> MR. W: Yeah. I've always worried that if I really allowed myself more power, I'd walk all over everybody.
>
> THERAPIST: I think we need to help you more with this feeling, particularly because it is so inhibiting and your behavior is so clearly at odds with your fears.

Reaction Formation

Reaction formation is the defense mechanism employed when patients cope with a frightening or disavowed feeling by turning it into its opposite. Although the mechanism is possibly more commonly found in patients with panic disorder, patients with depression also use it (Busch et al. 1995). Typically, the therapist observes depressed patients turning anger into a positive or helpful feeling, but some patients may convert guilt-provoking loving feelings into hatred. Although reaction formation is intended to avoid threatening sexual or aggressive feelings and fantasies, it usually intensifies underlying aggression over time, because patients cannot directly address the issues about which they are distressed. Depression emerges as the anger ultimately is directed inward. The therapist can help patients apprehend the presence of reaction formation by noting how the loving feelings they emphasize seem incongruous in the light of the problems they are discussing in the relationship.

Case Example 5

Ms. KK, a 24-year-old public relations consultant, became involved with Bob, who was quite needful of her support, as he was depressed because of losing his job and having financial woes. She expressed significant concerns about the relationship because she had a pattern of becoming involved with men who were dependent on her and then becoming frustrated and disappointed with them. When the therapist explored what attracted the patient to Bob in spite of his problems, Ms. KK focused on her boyfriend's positive traits, including his intelligence, congeniality, and warmth.

Over time, however, the boyfriend's dependency intensified. He moved in with the patient because of his financial difficulties and spent much of his time "hanging out" at her apartment, doing little in the way of housework. Ms. KK began to get increasingly depressed. She felt exhausted by Bob's problems, even though she felt she still needed to help him. She also became very critical with herself about her tendency to get involved with needy men. However, she expressed little direct anger toward him.

> THERAPIST: It seems like you would be more frustrated with Bob! It sounds as if he's really not doing much to earn his keep.
>
> MS. KK: He just really needs help. The problem's mine for getting involved with guys like this. I've got to try to understand more about that.
>
> THERAPIST: I certainly agree with you, but how do you feel about how he's conducting his life at this point?
>
> MS. KK: Well, I guess he could be doing more to help out me and himself. He's not looking for a job, but he could at least clean up the dishes. I mean, I'm supporting him.
>
> THERAPIST: Have you spoken to him about this?
>
> MS. KK: Well, some. But I don't want to get him even more upset. He really feels bad about himself.

Further exploration of the patient's pull toward needy men proved to be of value. Ms. KK's father was distant and critical, a successful entrepreneur who showed little emotion. She described her mother, on the other hand, as emotionally more connected to her, although acknowledging that she was also rather self-involved and somewhat depressed. Ms. KK seemed to feel that when she was needed by others, her attachment would be closer and more intimate. She feared getting angry because she worried that the man might be "sensitive" like her mother and feel injured, disrupting their tie. However, she became demoralized when she felt she was not getting what she needed from her relationships, including sexually.

As the work on this issue continued, Ms. KK became increasingly aware of her frustration. She decided that she needed to take some action, so she pressed her boyfriend to get a job and find his own place. To her surprise, he responded positively to these suggestions. As he became more independent, their satisfaction with the relationship increased.

References

Bloch AL, Shear MK, Markowitz JC, et al: An empirical study of defense mechanisms in dysthymia. Am J Psychiatry 150(8):1194–1198, 1993 8328563

Brenner C: Affects and psychic conflict. Psychoanal Q 44(1):5–28, 1975 1114198

Busch FN, Shear MK, Cooper AM, et al: An empirical study of defense mechanisms in panic disorder. J Nerv Ment Dis 183(5):299–303, 1995 7745383

Jacobson E: Depression: Comparative Studies of Normal, Neurotic, and Psychotic Conditions. New York, International Universities Press, 1971

11

The Termination Phase

Deciding to Terminate

Through an affectively charged relationship with the therapist, and through understanding gained in the interpretive work of the middle phase, patients gradually become 1) less vulnerable to loss, disappointment, and criticism; 2) capable of greater modulation of their feelings; 3) less guilty and self-punishing; and 4) capable of more realistic assessments of their own behaviors and motivations and those of others (Table 11–1). When patient and therapist feel that these improvements have become consistently incorporated into the individual's repertoire for dealing with stressful situations, thereby reducing vulnerability to recurrent depression, they may decide to end the treatment (Gaskill 1980; Tyson 1996; Weinshel 1992). An exception to this approach may be found in some brief structured psychodynamic treatments, which set a termination date after a limited number of sessions (Busch and Milrod 2015; Vinnars et al. 2013).

Often, patients, rather than the therapist, are first to bring up thoughts about ending therapy, which are explored to determine whether they are based on a realistic assessment of achievements made during treatment or represent a resistance to further work. It is useful at this point for therapist and patient to review the progress they have made in reducing depressive symptoms and helping the patient handle depressive feelings differently when they reemerge in new contexts. The general criteria presented in this chapter can provide a guide for assessing progress and readiness for entering the termination phase. When patient and therapist agree that significant and durable achievements have been made in treating depressed feelings, anticipat-

Table 11–1. Criteria for termination

1. Patient is less vulnerable to depression in the face of loss, disappointments, and criticism.
2. Patient can consistently better manage depressive feelings and aggression.
3. Patient is less prone to guilt and self-devaluation.
4. Patient can make more realistic assessments of own behavior and motivations and of those of others.

ing and managing situations in which they are likely to recur, they choose a date for termination. Enough time should be allowed in this phase to accomplish an understanding of the meaning and feelings about the loss of the therapeutic relationship.

The Process of Termination

During the termination phase, the therapeutic work focuses on the patient's feelings of narcissistic injury in relation to fantasies of a continued personal relationship with the therapist, feelings of loss and sadness about the ending of this important relationship, and anger toward the therapist regarding the termination or the limitations of treatment accomplishments. A recrudescence of symptoms is sometimes seen as the patient contends with feelings of loss, rejection, and/or anger (Firestein 1978).

Working with these feelings in patients who have already made considerable progress through treatment results in their increasing capacity to cope with loss and narcissistic injury, to direct their anger more effectively, and to show diminished guilt and self-punishment. This is accomplished by the thorough, emotionally charged exploration of the feelings and fantasies of loss, rejection, and reactive anger about ending the therapeutic relationship. Assisting patients to articulate what they have gained in treatment, juxtaposed against what they feel they are losing by ending the professional relationship, is often a helpful and moving experience (Firestein 1978; Tyson 1996).

Case Example 1

Ms. LL was a married writer in her late 50s who was born in Europe as World War II was ending. Her parents had been devastated by the effects of the war and seemed ill equipped to handle a serious medical condition that was diagnosed during her first year of life. Ms. LL spent two long periods in the hospital during her early years for treatment of this illness and was sent by her parents to a foster home each time she was discharged, because they felt unable to cope with the demands of her recuperation. When she was 10 years old, her mother separated from the family, after years of bitter fighting with her husband. Ms. LL was left in her father's care.

Ms. LL, who had dysthymia and generalized anxiety disorder, had experienced several episodes of moderate to severe depression in adulthood. She was again significantly depressed when she entered this psychodynamic treatment. Much of the therapy focused on her idealization of the distant, beautiful mother for whom she longed but whom she deeply resented, her bitter anger and constant expectation of rejection, her guilt about her "nasty pessimism," and her feelings of inadequacy as a woman to keep others engaged with her. Her difficult, rather depriving relationship with her husband was also a focus for the treatment.

After several years of therapy, Ms. LL was noticeably more successful and expressive in her work; much less guilty about her dealings with others, including her husband; and considerably less angry and embittered. As she became less accusatory and frustrated about her husband's difficulties with intimacy, their relationship greatly improved as well. She had not been significantly depressed for some time and had been able to understand and limit minor downturns in her mood successfully. Ms. LL and her therapist discussed her decision to terminate by reviewing her accomplishments in treatment and her concerns and fantasies about ending it. After spending some time on this discussion, and in the context of setting a termination date, her therapist revealed that in 6 months, she herself would be moving from the area.

At first Ms. LL handled this news matter-of-factly, expressing her gratitude and her curiosity about the reasons for the relocation. "I would have been ending anyway," she said, "so for once, this works out just right for me."

As time went on, however, she could acknowledge her anger and distress about what she experienced as her abandonment by the therapist.

> MS. LL: I've been depressed lately. And you—*you* are the reason! *I was the one leaving you*, and then you decided to leave me instead. Just like my mother! I don't think I can forgive you for that.
>
> THERAPIST: You feel as if when I go, I will be leaving you alone to deal with your husband and your illness all by yourself, just as she left you to deal with your difficult father and your condition all on your own.
>
> MS. LL [*crying*]: Yes! Of course, I know that it's different now. I really do feel better about handling things. But it's hard to shake these feelings. And I feel terrible about being so angry at you.
>
> THERAPIST: Before, you felt that your mother left *because* you were such a difficult child.

MS. LL: Yes, and I don't want to be difficult, especially now. I want you to have good feelings about me. But I also feel so disappointed that after all we've done and everything that's gotten better, I still feel like I'm stuck in a hard situation with my health. I'm not as successful as I would like to be, either. I don't want to seem ungrateful, but I think that if I were more famous, you would think more about me when you go.

THERAPIST: Yes, you always felt that being famous would get your parents' attention and show them that you weren't this sick, damaged person! You are really afraid that that's how I'll think about you, too.

MS. LL: I *have* learned to enjoy my career more—I really can get more pleasure from it now. I don't feel the same pressure to become famous and show everyone! I hope that doesn't change, because always wanting to be perfect and grab everyone's attention was just too much.

This vignette illustrates the mobilization of previous reactions to loss during the termination phase. It is valuable for the patient to experience these feelings and fantasies once again with the therapist, in this new treatment context. The termination period allows time for new material about the reactions to loss or rejection to emerge and be worked with, as well as for an emotionally laden reprise of previous work. It is often enormously reassuring for the patient to experience these familiar feelings while appreciating at the same time hard-won capacities to cope with them differently.

Handling Premature Requests for Termination

If the therapist believes that a request for termination is premature, it is important to articulate what further work may remain. This may include addressing the patient's guilty reactions in greater depth, exploring further a persistent tendency to idealize and devalue with destructive consequences, or continuing work on problems the patient may have in managing feelings of sadness, rejection, or anger. If the therapist feels that it is too early to end the treatment, an exploration of why the patient may be pulling away from their ongoing work is often quite helpful, in addition to the articulation by the therapist about the areas that require further exploration. Sometimes, such premature requests for termination may be based on dissatisfaction with treatment, such as the wish for a more structured approach, or may signal transference feelings that have been unaddressed. Exploring the patient's thoughts about termination in such cases may actually clarify obstacles to further progress or may establish trust that the therapist is sincere in the desire to be a coinvestigator of the patient's experience.

It is always advisable that therapists scan their own responses at such a juncture to be sure that countertransference wishes or extratherapeutic needs are not interfering with this judgment. For example, financial motivations or therapists' own abandonment fears may intrude on the decision to "let go" of patients with whom there is a good alliance. Further, therapists' own issues of perfectionism may be interfering with the assessment: patients may feel quite satisfied with their growth through the treatment, whereas therapists may have more demanding expectations (Gaskill 1980; Ticho 1972).

Sometimes, despite a therapist's feeling that more might be accomplished, patients insist on ending treatment. It is important at such a time to emphasize the importance of a termination phase to truly consolidate treatment gains. Often such patients will agree to further exploration if a termination date is set that allows some time to understand the impact of ending treatment. Depressive symptoms may recur during termination, and at such times, patients desiring a premature end to their treatment may recognize that they are having difficulties in managing this recurrence that could benefit from further therapy. One such patient, Ms. HH in Chapter 9 ("Idealization and Devaluation"), could acknowledge a significant problem with excessive alcohol use that she had previously denied during the treatment. When her depressive symptoms returned during a "trial termination" and precipitated a drinking binge, she finally felt able to appreciate the extent of her addiction and to explore it. She could better understand previously hidden dynamics through this work, preparing the way for an eventual, more successful termination.

At other times, patients may remain quite satisfied with the partial successes gained in therapy, and resistant to further exploration, because of unconscious fears about what might be exposed. Such patients may terminate therapy and then return later, when additional symptoms present. For instance, one man's incapacitating depression was considerably relieved with therapy, but when the treatment began to approach homosexual fantasies that made him feel guilty, disgusted with himself, and very anxious, he decided to terminate therapy. During the termination phase, the patient could acknowledge his awareness that further work might be helpful at some future point. When he returned to treatment several years later, he had successfully managed the occasional emergence of mild depressive symptoms without their escalating. He was quite anxious and having panic attacks, however, which fully resolved when he was able to understand more about the fantasies that had been avoided earlier. In a follow-up phone call several years after this second treatment, the man reported being largely free of depressive and anxiety symptoms.

Countertransference Reactions During the Termination Phase

Common countertransference feelings at the time of termination include guilt about ending the treatment, reflecting the patient's, and sometimes the therapist's, experience of it as an abandonment. Feelings of uncertainty and inadequacy about the therapy's effectiveness may also emerge, often reflecting the patient's renewed struggles with idealization and devaluation under the pressure of a final assessment of accomplishments. It is important for the therapist to reflect on the origins and meanings of these feelings within the treatment context and to ensure that the patient's concerns in these areas are vigorously explored (Tyson 1996).

Case Example 2

Ms. MM was a 37-year-old single travel agent who had masochistic tendencies and moderately severe depression when she presented for psychotherapy. Over the course of a several-year treatment, she came to understand a good deal about her depressions and about her masochistic style of interaction with others. Ms. MM had initially chosen lovers and friends who were charismatic and lively like her father, a banker who gambled, had affairs, and drank to excess, only to be as disappointed in their inattentiveness to her needs as she had been in his. She secretly identified with her friends' exuberance and charisma and continually effaced herself, which her very depressed mother typically had done with her father. "Sometimes I feel like the piece of dirt that sticks to your shoe," she would say, early in treatment. "I feel like I'm a mess—I don't think I deserve these relationships and I just freeze in them. I can't show people who I really am, and then I get so sad and upset when they don't figure it out! It just makes me feel all that much more worthless."

One of the things that Ms. MM eventually identified as most helpful in her treatment was the fact that her therapist "got" her—she felt understood and could then understand many aspects of her own feelings, thoughts, and behaviors. Early in the treatment, she also tested whether the therapist cared enough to actually "come after" her, by, for instance, missing a session or two and not calling. After the therapist called to inquire about her absence, they discussed this wish to be cared for. They also eventually discussed the provocative and aggressive elements of her behavior, and the patient began to see how sometimes she provoked abandonment by inexplicably withdrawing from others.

Ms. MM made considerable gains in her treatment, eventually being promoted several times in her agency, as she felt better able to demonstrate her significant organizational abilities. She also married a man who was deeply caring and supportive. Her mother died during the course of her therapy, and Ms. MM could grieve and fully understand the depth of both her love and her frustration for her mother.

When she eventually discussed her thoughts about termination, it was with some trepidation. "My husband thinks that I am ready, but I'm not so sure. I'm not going to do it for him. I want to be really clear that I am doing this for *me*. He does understand a lot about me, but in ending our therapy, I'll be losing you, and I think you still understand me better than almost anyone."

With continued discussion of termination over the next weeks, Ms. MM felt increasingly sure about the decision, with which her therapist concurred, and a date was set 5 months away, just before the therapist's customary summer vacation and the time at which Ms. MM and her husband were also planning to travel. In the week following this decision, however, Ms. MM became quietly very sad. "The date we picked is pretty near my mother's birthday, and I think I will feel really alone. She wasn't able to connect with me the way you do, and now you will be gone, too. I'm not sure that I'm really ready for this if I feel so sad."

Her therapist briefly considered changing the termination date because of this information, but then reconsidered. She realized that she would be making the change largely out of a guilty wish to protect Ms. MM from the sad feelings she was inevitably experiencing about the treatment's end and from transient doubts about the adequacy of the treatment, which in this case reflected her patient's fears, rather than her own assessment of the case. She knew that Ms. MM still struggled in subtle ways with a guilty tendency to negate her progress. Although the therapist knew that the patient would feel sad about termination, she also thought that she was emphasizing her sense of loss and abandonment at the expense of considering her happiness about her achievements—her loving marriage and the new promotion that enabled her to take a very exciting vacation that year. She realized that exploring Ms. MM's feelings would be the best way to determine whether the decision had been a sound one. She asked Ms. MM if she could talk more about her feelings of sadness.

> MS. MM: Well, I feel bittersweet, really. I do feel so happy about everything I've done here, everything I've learned about myself. I guess I'm still worried that all that will dissolve in some strange way the minute I'm out of your sight.
>
> THERAPIST: That sounds familiar, doesn't it?

MS. MM: Yes! I know that I felt that way when my mother was so
depressed those times. I really didn't feel safe—I was so worried about her. I guess *she* was the one who seemed to be dis-
solving. But that made me feel so alone, like I could just
disappear, too. My dad wasn't involved enough with any of
us to even notice what was going on with me! I don't know
if he even realized how depressed she was! She would sort of
pull it together a little more for him.
THERAPIST: Do you think that might have something to do with
why you don't entirely trust that your husband will help you
feel less terribly alone when we end our therapy?
MS. MM: Duh! Yes, of course. But I do still feel sad.
THERAPIST: I know. You've felt so close to me, and you're worried
about where all those feelings will go.
MS. MM: I guess I know that you will always be a part of my life
that I carry around inside me, but right now that just doesn't
feel like enough! I carried around what I could of each of my
parents, too, but it didn't add up to enough, ever. [*Tearfully*]
Well, things make so much more sense now, and I do feel
more whole. But I'll just really miss you...this office, your
smile. I don't have much reason to come back to this neighborhood after we finish, but I think I might now and then,
just to see it. Or maybe I won't want to—I don't know.

As the months passed, Ms. MM could talk about her sadness in a
deeply heartfelt way, and about her anger that her relationship with her
therapist would change in some irrevocable way once she no longer came
to see her twice a week. She did not become depressed, however, as she had
feared. Two months before her termination date, the patient unexpectedly
did not come to one of her sessions and called to acknowledge this only
after a few hours had passed. Because this was now quite unusual behavior,
her therapist had considered calling the patient before finally receiving
Ms. MM's call. She decided, however, that this impulse was based on a
feeling of wanting to reassure her patient that the therapist still cared and
was concerned, more than out of any real concern on her part, and decided
to wait to explore the behavior in their next session.

MS. MM: I'm really sorry that I didn't call you. I was at my doctor's
office, and he sent me over for an X ray, and it all took much
longer than I realized. I could have probably called from my
cell phone, but somehow I didn't realize that I had it with
me until I finally saw it in my purse and called you.
THERAPIST: Do you think anything else might have been going on?
MS. MM: Well, it did remind me of those times in the beginning
when I didn't come to session and didn't call to cancel. I know
we thought it was because I was testing to see if you even no-

ticed or cared. Maybe, in a way, there was something like that now. Being at the doctor always makes me feel a little nervous, and the thought that I needed an X ray did make me wonder what it would be like to go through something without having you right here to talk about it with. Maybe I was angry and punishing you, and also just testing—to be sure you still cared or would be worried about me. Or if knowing that I'm doing better means that you won't think about me, about how I am doing.

THERAPIST: Do you really think that after all these years, I wouldn't think about you?

MS. MM: No, I'm sure that you will. But it helps to hear you say it!

THERAPIST: I think that you did feel that the only way you could get through to your mother, especially when she was depressed, was to try to get her to notice that something was wrong. It feels scary that maybe you won't be cared for and thought about when everything is okay!

This case example illustrates the importance of therapists' examining their own reactions to determine whether they represent either a sound clinical judgment or a countertransference response elicited by patients' feelings or by the therapists' own reactions to the termination. Once therapists explore such personal feelings and address within therapy any behaviors by patients that may provoke such a reassessment, they usually can determine whether new material is emerging that may change the recommendation to terminate.

The decision to terminate is one arrived at mutually between therapist and patient, when enduring progress is judged to have been made. The accomplishments of treatment have allowed the patient to become consistently less guilty, better able to manage and understand depressive feelings, and considerably less self-devaluing. Strong feelings about abandonment or about the loss of an idealized relationship often come to the fore in depressed patients during the termination phase and allow for an affectively charged and moving exploration that strengthens the accomplishments already made within therapy. Therapists should be particularly alert to countertransference reactions common to this treatment phase.

References

Busch FN, Milrod BL: Psychodynamic treatment for separation anxiety in a treatment nonresponder. J Am Psychoanal Assoc 63(5):893–919, 2015 26487108

Firestein S: Termination in Psychoanalysis. New York, International Universities Press, 1978

Gaskill HS: The closing phase of the psychoanalytic treatment of adults and the goals of psychoanalysis 'The myth of perfectibility'. Int J Psychoanal 61(1):11–23, 1980 7364534

Ticho EA: Termination of psychoanalysis: treatment goals, life goals. Psychoanal Q 41(3):315–333, 1972 5047036

Tyson P: Termination of psychoanalysis and psychotherapy, in Textbook of Psychoanalysis. Edited by Nersessian E, Kopff RG Jr. Washington, DC, American Psychiatric Press, 1996, pp 501–524

Vinnars B, Frydman Dixon S, Barber JP: Pragmatic psychodynamic psychotherapy—bridging contemporary psychoanalytic clinical practice and evidence-based psychodynamic practice. Psychoanal Inq 33:567–583, 2013

Weinshel EM: Therapeutic technique in psychoanalysis and psychoanalytic psychotherapy. J Am Psychoanal Assoc 40(2):327–347, 1992 1593075

III PART

Special Topics

12

CHAPTER

Psychodynamic Approaches to Depression With Comorbid Personality Disorder

AS noted in Chapter 1 ("Introduction"), depressive and personality disorders have a high rate of comorbidity (37.9% in a major epidemiological study; Hasin et al. 2005). In addition, comorbid personality disorders adversely affect treatment outcome, reducing adherence and response (American Psychiatric Association 2013). The most common disorders that co-occur are Cluster C personality disorders, including avoidant, dependent, and obsessive-compulsive personality disorders (Corruble et al. 1996; Friborg et al. 2014). For the most part the presence of Cluster C personality disorders does not require major changes from the techniques described in this book, because there is an overlap in symptomatology and dynamics between these personality disorders and depression. Patients with these disorders often experience guilt and fears about angry feelings and fantasies that can become self-directed, the typical dynamics of depression cycle 1 (see Chapter 2, "Development of a Psychodynamic Model of Depression"). However, as described below, these disorders can benefit from particular emphases on relevant key personality factors. Depression may also occur with Cluster B personality disorders (Corruble et al. 1996; Friborg et al. 2014). In this chapter we discuss comorbid borderline and narcissistic personality disorders, which typically require a more significant modification of psychodynamic approaches to depression.

Dependent and Avoidant Personality Disorders

In patients with dependent personality disorder, therapists make an effort to identify dependent feelings and fantasies. These can include a belief of being unable to function effectively alone, which is often at odds with the patient's actual capabilities, and fears of losing or damaging needed others. A chronic sense of inadequacy and narcissistic humiliation can accompany these high levels of dependency. Underlying conflicts include a fear of disruption from angry feelings and fantasies toward significant attachment figures upon whom the patient feels dependent. Fearfulness of losing a needed attachment figure inhibits direct expression of anger, disagreement, or self-assertion. In these instances anger can become self-directed, leading to guilt and self-critical feelings. Helping patients to confront fantasies of their own inadequacy and fragility in their relationships can help them to feel less dependent and safer experiencing angry feelings and experimenting with more assertive behaviors.

Dependency frequently exacerbates a tendency to idealize others, permitting a feeling of protection and safety. These idealized perceptions in turn heighten the fantasy that the other person is necessary for self-esteem or safety. The perception of an idealized other affects the patient's realistic perception of the self, as the self is devalued in comparison to a powerful other, heightening feelings of inadequacy (depression cycle 2). Idealization is perforce threatened by disappointments with the attachment figure, adding to unconscious conflicted anger. Identifying the tendency toward idealization can help patients to develop a more realistic perception of the capabilities of the self in relation to others, helping to diminish their feelings of inadequacy and reduce recurrent disappointments.

Avoidant personality disorder is also closely intertwined with depressive dynamics. Patients with avoidant personality disorder are described in the DSM-5 (American Psychiatric Association 2013) as having "feelings of inadequacy, and hypersensitivity to negative evaluation..." (p. 672), and such patients tend to avoid social situations that are associated with such feelings. These constellations suggest a high level of narcissistic vulnerability. In patients with comorbid avoidant personality disorder, depressive dynamics enhance fears of expressing anger or self-assertion due to anticipated rejection or criticism, potentially redirecting anger toward the self. With these patients it is useful to explore situations they are avoiding, and to identify the negative fantasies contributing to feelings of inadequacy and expected negative judgments. As their concerns are addressed, patients will often attempt to confront situations that they have avoided, providing an opportunity to directly assess fantasized feared outcomes. Although the dynamic therapist does not typically instruct patients to confront feared situations, the therapist can look at why patients are avoiding them and how they might address them. An example would be Mr. T's fear of confronting his wife about her withdrawal from their relationship (see Chapter 7, "Addressing Angry Reactions to Narcissistic Injury"). Although Mr. T felt inadequate and feared damaging their relationship, his confrontation of his wife lead to greater intimacy.

Obsessive-Compulsive Personality Disorder

The dynamic therapist should be alert to the various traits of obsessive-compulsive personality disorder when present, including a preoccupation with details, "perfectionism that interferes with task completion," excessive involvement with work, and inflexibility "about matters of morality, ethics, or values" (American Psychiatric Association 2013, p. 678). The preoccupation with work and details can be seen as defenses that allow the patient to avoid the experience of more intense feelings. It is of importance for the therapist to interpret these defenses over time, identifying feelings such as rejection fears, dependent longings or angry fantasies the patient may be keeping out of consciousness. Rigidity about morality and ethics suggests a severe superego that parallels depressive dynamics in many patients. These patients are often highly self-critical about their inability to meet self-expectations. The therapist seeks to identify whether a severe superego is present and how associated self-criticism and guilt may be contributing to depression.

Perfectionism can represent an effort to respond to the demands of a severe superego and a defense against the experience of certain feelings. This trait can also function as a compensatory self-idealization in response to feelings of inadequacy. However, perfectionism typically contributes to low self-esteem as patients feel pressured to meet unreasonable goals and expectations. Perfectionism and severe self-criticism have been found to be particularly difficult traits to address in treatment of depression. Blatt et al. (1995, 1998) reanalyzed data from the Treatment of Depression Collaborative Research Program (TDCRP; Elkin et al. 1989), which compared 16-week treatments with imipramine, once-weekly cognitive-behavioral therapy (CBT), once-weekly interpersonal psychotherapy (IPT), and clinical management (the "placebo" arm). There were no differences found between the three active treatments, with approximately 35% of the patients recovering (defined as minimal or no symptoms for at least 8 consecutive weeks after treatment termination). The additional analyses (Blatt et al. 1995, 1998) revealed that pretreatment perfectionism or self-criticism, as measured by the Dysfunctional Attitude Scale (DAS; Weissman and Beck 1978), independent of treatment condition, significantly diminished the reduction in depressive symptoms.

Blatt et al. (2010) concluded that patients with perfectionistic and highly self-critical tendencies may require longer-term psychotherapies to address these factors. These self-views are often embedded subconsciously and occur reflexively and may take many interventions to address effectively.

Case Example 1

Ms. NN, who suffered from a severe and persistent depression with intense self-criticism, was slow to reveal and recognize very high self-standards and perfectionistic tendencies. Although she had graduated from a prestigious business school, at age 32 she had yet to hold a job for an extended period and felt she could not even accomplish small projects around the house. It emerged that she also believed that these tasks needed to be done perfectly. The therapist found that the patient had very high self-expectations, adding to an anticipation of failure.

> THERAPIST: Why can't you think about moving forward with your plan to clean the basement?
> Ms. NN: Because I'll fail. I've never really accomplished anything.
> THERAPIST: What about completing business school?
> Ms. NN: Well, that didn't really mean anything. I wasn't really near the top of the class. And I didn't get selected at the best internships.
> THERAPIST: Well let me try to understand that. If you're not at the top of the class or selected at an excellent internship instead of a top one, then that's a failure?
> Ms. NN: Well you have to have some standards. Why don't we just say "Oh great for you. You also graduated from high school."
> THERAPIST: I think your standards and expectations may be much

> higher than you recognize. I think this makes it much more difficult for you to achieve something that you are satisfied with. It both makes you more wary of even trying and more self-critical of efforts you do make.
>
> Ms. NN: Well I don't know. These standards make sense to me.

Ms. NN's perfectionism and high standards were so ingrained, and her self-condemnation so automatic, that it took many clarifications on the part of the therapist for her to identify and acknowledge these tendencies.

According to Blatt et al. (2010), the role of perfectionism and self-criticism can be segregated in therapeutic responsiveness. He and his colleagues (Blatt and Shohar 2013) described two forms of depression, one deriving primarily from problems in relationships with others (*dependent*) and one related to efforts at autonomy and self-control (*introjective*). Dependent depressed patients, in this view, are characterized by loneliness, fears of abandonment and aggression, idealization of others, and impulsivity. Patients with introjective depression demonstrate guilt, shame, worthlessness, self-criticism, fear of disapproval, and hypermorality. Our approach emphasizes the interrelatedness of these dynamics, and we have found that many patients are better characterized as "mixed" types. For example, patients with dependent depression may be highly self-critical because they believe that certain traits will cause them to be rejected; and patients with introjective depression may be preoccupied with possible rejection based on their own negative self-judgments (others would not want to be with them due to aspects of their personalities about which they feel shame and guilt). In the psychodynamic treatment we recommend, the clinician should be alert to the various symptoms, character traits, and dynamics that emerge with a given patient and attend to those appropriately.

Narcissistic and Borderline Personality Disorders

Comorbid narcissistic or borderline personality disorder and depressive disorders require some modification in treatment. According to the DSM-5 (American Psychiatric Association 2013), narcissistic personality disorder is characterized by patients' views of themselves as superior, often exaggerating their achievements, and expectations that others recognize and admire their talents. They may be preoccupied with fantasies about success and power. Patients typically have a sense of entitlement and expect special favors or treatment from others. The disorder can be accompanied by an inability or unwillingness to recognize the needs and feelings of others. Patients are often envious of others and believe others envy them.

Although DSM-5 emphasizes feelings of superiority or entitlement in these patients, these symptoms frequently occur in the context of a severe form of narcissistic vulnerability. Patients with low self-esteem can easily feel disregarded and rejected—feelings that are often suppressed. Frequently their dynamics are related to disappointment in their expectations of responsiveness and admiration. They may become enraged at and devaluing of people who do not recognize their specialness, with a compensatory idealization of others whom they view as linked to or cognizant of their specialness. Frequent anger at and disappointment and limited empathy with others causes disruption of their close relationships. As noted in Chapter 9 ("Idealization and Devaluation"), some patients with narcissistic personality disorder require concrete representations, such as material objects, as evidence of their self-worth and can become depressed when they do not obtain these tokens.

A key issue in treating such patients is that they usually do not recognize their level of expectations or their narcissistic tendencies. They typically respond angrily if someone points out their excessive expectations or entitlement. In an effort to engage patients in treatment, the therapist can explore the circumstances in which the patient feels disappointed, as well as rage at others for not adequately recognizing their capabilities or responding to their demands. Therapists help patients to recognize their underlying narcissistic vulnerability and low self-esteem and the efforts to manage their self-esteem through idealized self-views and expectations of others. In addition to relieving depressive vulnerability by addressing these narcissistic dynamics, a depressive episode, and the circumstances surrounding its onset, often provide greater access to underlying feelings of low self-esteem and disappointment.

Case Example 2

Mr. OO, a highly successful lawyer, decided to leave his law practice to join a startup developing a legal services software program. However, this new line of work was disappointing and frustrating for him. He was angry with the founders of the firm for not giving him adequate credit for his legal knowledge and for not providing him a role that was commensurate with his view of his capacities. Clashes erupted as he demanded more executive tasks and more money. He was told that although his knowledge was important, he did not have adequate programming skills or knowledge to play the role he hoped for. He decided to leave the company with a plan to return to his old firm, but unexpectedly, at least in his view, the firm was not interested. At this point he became severely depressed and sought treatment. His symptoms partially responded to a trial of venlafaxine as the therapist explored his reactions to his circumstances.

> MR. OO: I didn't realize that the founders of the firm were such idiots. Their plan turned out to be pie in the sky and the firm is still struggling. If they had listened to my practical advice, they would already have a product worth selling.
> THERAPIST: I realize their behavior was terribly disappointing to you, and it was even more shocking when your old firm did not want you back.
> MR. OO: Well, that's what's really stupid. You would think they would realize how much money they would make from me like they did before.
> THERAPIST: Do you have any idea what happened?
> MR. OO: Well, I'm surrounded by idiots who don't think practically, who don't know how to pursue a business opportunity. But now I feel like such an idiot. I misjudged other people's capacities and look where it's landed me. Now I think no other firm is going to be interested in me. I'm damaged goods.

Rather than his typical railing against others, Mr. OO was more preoccupied with viewing himself as a failure. He had not applied for other jobs, with the expectation they would not be interested, even when other colleagues told him that given his capabilities it would not be difficult to find comparable employment. But he responded that then he would be at a second-rate firm and lose the respect of others in his area of expertise. He had dreams in which he was excluded from meetings of his old law partners and felt lost and alone. He believed it was unfair that this had happened to him based on others who did not recognize his talents.

In exploring Mr. OO's background it emerged that both parents were quite judgmental and critical of him. His father was very demanding with regard to his performance in sports and often complained that he was lazy. From early on Mr. OO had the feeling that nothing would satisfy his mother's expectations, and over the course of therapy he concluded that she may have been depressed. He struggled with sports but was recognized for his academic skills, although this did not seem to change his parents' criticism. He developed a smugness and arrogance about his academic capacities, which increased after his acceptance at a prestigious university and law school. Currently, both parents were unempathic when it came to the pain surrounding his job loss, pressing him to "stop messing around and find work."

THERAPIST: It does seem as if your parents have always judged you critically. It's no wonder that your academic and job success became so important to you.

MR. OO: Athletics was embarrassing to me and my father. It seemed liked my skills were finally being recognized when people realized I was smart. Now I'm back to being with idiots.

THERAPIST: I'm wondering whether the people at your startup and firm remind you of your parents, and this increases the very negative feelings you've had when they criticize you.

MR. OO: Hmm…Those feelings might be connected. These firms really don't get my talents, just like my parents, and they're going to suffer for that.

Here the therapist has allied with Mr. OO in looking at his underlying narcissistic vulnerability and his anger. The therapist also began to work with Mr. OO on his refusal to consider a "second-rate" firm as his unemployment was only adding to his depression. He eventually obtained a new job, although he demeaned it. The therapist made efforts to address Mr. OO's alienation of others through his arrogance or over-expectation as problems emerged in his new firm, where he believed the work and people were inferior. The therapist tactfully introduced the idea that his anger at others and how it was expressed might end up alienating them.

MR. OO: So the people in this work group are just not good. I made suggestions to them that were very valuable and they rejected them, asking me to come up with a different plan. I'm not going to work with idiots and I told the leader of the group that.

THERAPIST: And how did he respond?

MR. OO: Not well. He said that they would have to think about reevaluating my contract. But I don't think they will. I'm having too much success in my area.

THERAPIST: We've talked about how hurt and angry you feel when you experience others as not recognizing or getting you. But I think because you feel so strongly that sometimes it makes it hard for you to step back and consider how best to express your feelings. Your responses can hurt and anger others.

MR. OO: I guess I realize that on some level. But I find working with these people intolerable.

At this point the therapist explored with Mr. OO what felt intolerable in these circumstances, with some movement in helping him to identify that feelings and reactions that added to his negative self-view and interpersonal conflicts. He was able to reduce his criticisms of himself and his colleagues regarding his new job.

Despite the progress demonstrated in this case, it is important to note that narcissistic personality traits are deeply embedded and can take extended effort to relieve. Unfortunately many such patients will leave treatment or opt for medication management once their depression has lifted, because they tend to feel misunderstood by the therapist (e.g., the therapist does not recognize others are to blame or the patient is entitled to special treatment), or not see the value of further exploration.

Borderline personality disorder is described in DSM-5 (American Psychiatric Association 2013, p. 663) as "a pervasive pattern of instability of interpersonal relationships, self-image, and affects, and marked impulsivity" as indicated by at least five of the following: "frantic efforts to avoid real or imagined abandonment," "a pattern of unstable and intense interpersonal relationships characterized by alternating between extremes of idealization and devaluation," "identity disturbance: markedly and persistently unstable self-image or sense of self," "impulsivity...," "recurrent suicidal behavior, gestures, or threats, or self-mutilating behavior," "affective instability due to a marked reactivity of mood," "chronic feelings of emptiness," "inappropriate intense anger or difficulty controlling anger," and "transient, stress-related paranoid ideation or severe dissociative symptoms." Depressive disorders frequently co-occur with borderline personality disorder.

This book does not provide formal methods to approach patients with borderline personality disorder, for whom a number of treatments have been developed and tested, including dialectical behavior therapy, transference-focused psychotherapy, and mentalization-based therapy (Olds and Busch 2014). However, it is important in the treatment of depression to be alert to the presence of borderline personality, as the disorder must be addressed and may be the primary psychopathology, with depression emerging secondarily. Thus, methods and approaches that aid patients in developing mentalization skills, recognizing their distorted perception of others as all good or all bad, and managing their rage are of value.

Kernberg's (1967) model of borderline personality disorder clearly delineates the dynamics of patients with borderline personality, allowing an understanding of how these dynamics interact with those of depressive disorders. He posited that these patients, who are usually insecurely attached, are unable to modulate and tolerate negative affects, such as rage or envy, and fear, often unconsciously, that they will destroy a needed "good object." The split perception of others is a defensive reaction to this danger, as rage is experienced toward those who are already devalued and kept separate from others who are idealized attachment figures. However, these defenses interfere with the development of more complex views of self and others and a more consolidated identify that can aid in better regulation of negative emotions. In addition, these idealizations and devaluations are fluid, as an "all good" object can suddenly become "all bad." Transference-focused psychotherapy (Yeomans et al. 2015), based on this model, provides an opportunity to address these split and shifting self and other representations as they emerge with the therapist, helping to clarify and manage the intolerable feelings and defensive splitting.

In depressed borderline patients, poorly managed anger can readily become self-directed in the form of severe self-criticism and suicidality. In addition, patients can become depressed from not having a sense of a secure attachment figure, and from recurrent disruptions in relationships related to poor impulse control and poor management and expression of rage. The dynamics of idealization of others leading to disappointment and devaluation (depression cycle 2) are prominent. Thus, helping patients to develop a greater capacity for mentalization, to better manage their rage, and to recognize and understand their propensity to split others into all good and all bad interdigitate with addressing depressive dynamics. Ultimately a broader and more variegated understanding and perception of others can help to ease anger, depression, and interpersonal conflicts.

Case Example 3

Ms. PP, a 48-year-old divorced lawyer who presented with periods of severe depression, struggled with intense and unstable relationships, shifting idealization and devaluation of others, intense bouts of rage and affective instability, abandonment fears, impulsivity, and suicidality. She felt isolated and frustrated after her divorce and recurrent disruptions in relationships with friends triggered by conflicts about their not being more helpful to her during her divorce. She was not working as a lawyer and had identity struggles concerning what career she should pursue. She was very involved with her family but would feel depressed, frustrated, and anxious after spending time with them. She would shift from viewing her mother as exploitative, controlling, and help-rejecting, to a sense of her as legitimately needing help, a victim of her alcoholic father's harsh criticism and treatment. When Ms. PP viewed her mother as a victim, she felt guilty about not doing more for her. She felt pressured to "rescue" her mother, but after spending time with her at her parents' house, she became enraged at her mother's unwillingness to listen or make efforts on her own behalf. Additionally, Ms. PP was criticized by her father, who would refer to her as mentally ill and useless, triggering hurt and rage, followed by a depressed mood and suicidal threats. When enraged at him, she claimed she would not visit home again. In the course of psychotherapy, after multiple unsuccessful medication trials, her treatment was aided by the use of an antipsychotic, quetiapine, and an antidepressant, sertraline, which provided limited easing of her symptoms.

The therapist helped Ms. PP identify a pattern in which she would meet others whom she initially viewed positively in terms of their efforts to be responsive to her. However, she would subsequently feel disappointed by them, experiencing them as either incompetent, or as having lied or taken advantage of her. At these points the patient felt there was nothing good about them, seeing them as very hurtful and damaging, and became intensely self-critical for not screening these relationships better.

When the cycle involving her family restarted and she planned to revisit home to help her mother, the therapist attempted to point out these shifting views and how she subsequently felt exploited. She would become enraged at the therapist for not understanding her mother and the patient's need to help her, providing an opportunity to explore these factors in the transference.

> MS. PP: I don't see why you don't get it. My mother desperately needs my help. I have to visit her.
> THERAPIST: Yes, but then afterward you become very depressed and frustrated with her.
> MS. PP: Well, that's because my father attacks me. He's a total jerk and he keeps her down.
> THERAPIST: I understand your feelings about him but you also get frustrated and disappointed with your mother. Then you get furious with yourself and very depressed.
> MS. PP: I forgot about that. But I have to go there. Right now I just feel guilty I don't spend enough time with her.

In a subsequent session the therapist worked with identifying the shift in her feelings toward him when gripped by her guilt.

> MS. PP: I really think I should quit treatment when you talk about reconsidering going home.
> THERAPIST: Well, I wonder if the same process goes on here as with your friends. You can find me very helpful, but then you become disappointed when I don't get you and become furious with me.
> MS. PP: I know we've discussed this pattern, but right now I think you just don't get it and I'm not sure I see the point in continuing.
> THERAPIST: I understand that, but events like this represent a chance to see that angry feelings can be dealt with in a different way from how your family handles them, and you could feel furious with me at one point and see me as quite helpful at another.

MS. PP: Well right now I'm not finding you too helpful. But I
know you have been.

In between the stormy periods Ms. PP became more agreeable at looking the way her feelings shifted, including in the transference. The therapist worked with her on identifying her shifting idealization and devaluations of others, her anger and disappointment, and her subsequent self-
criticism. Over time she came to recognize her harshly negative view of
others and of herself as her anger turned toward herself. She began to consider her own contribution to conflicts with others, and her fears of her
own anger being damaging. Another valuable tool for Ms. PP was mentalization, as she began to consider what others might be struggling with internally.

MS. PP: I know I shouldn't have gone home but I did do better
dealing with my father. I was thinking of the things we talked
about in his history.
THERAPIST: How did this help?
MS. PP: I realize he had to deal with his father suiciding. He grew
up with just his mother, who was often depressed and drinking. I think he's very angry and frightened about my mother
having problems and worried I might make things worse.
This doesn't excuse his behavior, but I understand it better.

These observations led her to a more complex view of others rather than
as all good or all bad, victims or victimizers. This helped to ease her feelings
of hurt and anger and to identify better ways she might interact with others.
Although her mood shifts and polarizations continued, the gradual modulation of these states helped over time to relieve her depression and borderline personality symptoms, and improve her relationships.

References

American Psychiatric Association: Diagnostic and Statistical Manual of Mental
Disorders, 5th Edition. Arlington, VA, American Psychiatric Association,
2013
Blatt SJ, Shohar G: A dialectic model of personality development and psychopa-
thology: recent contributions to understanding and treating depression, in A
Dialectic Model of Personality Development and Psychopathology: Recent
Contributions in the Theory and Treatment of Depression: Toward a Dy-
namic Interactionism Model. Edited by Corveleyn J, Luyten P, Blatt SJ. New
York, Routledge, 2013, pp 137–162

Blatt SJ, Quinlan DM, Pilkonis PA, Shea MT: Impact of perfectionism and need for approval on the brief treatment of depression: the National Institute of Mental Health Treatment of Depression Collaborative Research Program revisited. J Consult Clin Psychol 63(1):125–132, 1995 7896977

Blatt SJ, Zuroff DC, Bondi CM, et al: When and how perfectionism impedes the brief treatment of depression: Further analyses of the NIMH TDCRP. J Consult Clin Psychol 66:423–428, 1998 9583345

Blatt SJ, Zuroff DC, Hawley LL, Auerbach JS: Predictors of sustained therapeutic change. Psychother Res 20(1):37–54, 2010 19757328

Corruble E, Ginestet D, Guelfi JD: Comorbidity of personality disorders and unipolar major depression: a review. J Affect Disord 37(2-3):157–170, 1996 8731079

Elkin I, Shea MT, Watkins JT, et al: NIMH Treatment of Depression Collaborative Research Program: general effectiveness of treatments. Arch Gen Psychiatry 46:971–983, 1989 2684085

Friborg O, Martinsen EW, Martinussen M, et al: Comorbidity of personality disorders in mood disorders: a meta-analytic review of 122 studies from 1988 to 2010. J Affect Disord 152–154:1–11, 2014 24120406

Hasin DS, Goodwin RD, Stinson FS, Grant BF: Epidemiology of major depressive disorder: results from the National Epidemiologic Survey on Alcoholism and Related Conditions. Arch Gen Psychiatry 62(10):1097–1106, 2005 16203955

Kernberg O: Borderline personality organization. J Am Psychoanal Assoc 15(3):641–685, 1967 4861171

Olds DD, Busch FN: Psychotherapy, in Psychiatry, 3rd Edition. Edited by Cutler J. New York, Oxford University Press, 2014, pp 557-609

Weissman AN, Beck AT: Development and validation of the Dysfunctional Attitude Scale: a preliminary investigation. Paper presented at the 62nd Annual Meeting of the American Educational Research Association, Toronto, Ontario, Canada, March 27–31, 1978

Yeomans FE, Clarkin JF, Kernberg OF: Transference-Focused Psychotherapy for Borderline Personality Disorder: A Clinical Guide. Washington, DC, American Psychiatric Publishing, 2015

13

Managing Impasses and Negative Reactions to Treatment

PATIENTS with more severe and persistent depressive disorder represent a particular challenge for the psychodynamic psychotherapist. Certainly, when depressive symptoms are intense and not responding to treatment, it is important to make ongoing psychopharmacological efforts to reduce the level of depression. However, some patients continue to struggle with persistent depression in spite of these efforts.

In addition, a subset of patients experience therapy as an adverse, negative process. Although analysts tend to view therapy as a healing, supportive process, these patients can experience it as hurtful and damaging. In some instances, these patients drop out of treatment and constitute treatment "failures." It is therefore important to identify factors that may be disruptive to treatment and lead to a negative therapeutic reaction (Asch 1976; Freud 1923). Patients in whom improvement triggers guilt and guilt-driven disruptions to therapy are discussed in Chapter 9, "Idealization and Devaluation" (see the case of Mr. GG). Other factors that can contribute to impasses in treatment include significant impairments in patients' sense of basic trust, severe narcissistic sensitivity, a history of trauma, and a comorbid personality disorder (see Chapter 12, "Psychodynamic Approaches to Depression With Comorbid Personality Disorder"). In these cases, it is particularly important to find ways of strengthening the therapeutic alliance and affirming treatment goals.

189

Patients with such impairments often trigger countertransference reactions in the therapist, including helplessness and frustration, which if communicated to patients, could worsen symptoms. It is very important for the therapist to be alert to these feelings in these difficult cases; if recognized, they may provide valuable information about how to best approach these patients (see Case Example 1 below and the section "Working With Countertransference Feelings" in Chapter 5, "The Middle Phase of Treatment").

Impairments in Basic Trust

Some patients, often as a consequence of severe trauma or abuse, are chronically terrified that they will be damaged or rejected by others, and they lack a core feeling that others will try to help them. Such patients often expect that the therapist will be critical and rejecting of them as well. In more difficult cases, patients experience the therapist as behaving in hurtful and critical ways, even in the absence of therapeutic errors. In these cases, it is particularly important to attend to the therapeutic alliance. Whereas typically a therapeutic alliance with a sense of basic trust in the therapist as an ally is established in the first few sessions, with these patients the establishment of a trusting relationship is often a slow and painstaking process. Much effort is needed to help such patients feel that the therapist is an ally in efforts to understand and treat the depression, and, throughout treatment, it is often necessary to examine with patients why they may feel otherwise.

Case Example 1

Mr. QQ, a 36-year-old laboratory technician, grew up experiencing his mother as intensely critical of him and otherwise neglectful. He felt that his mother was very self-involved, was focused on her own appearance, and disregarded pressing emotional and physical needs of her children. Mr. QQ also felt that his mother favored the other children and that they were often allied as a team against him. Mr. QQ was close to his father, who, however, died when Mr. QQ was 10 years old. This left him feeling trapped with a critical family and no allies, and with conflicted anger at his father for abandoning him.

Mr. QQ was extremely fearful that his therapist would treat him in a critical and abandoning way, just as he had experienced in his family. In fact, a transference-countertransference enactment had occurred with his previous therapist in which the therapist said that she could no longer work with the patient after his hospitalization for a particularly severe bout of depression. Mr. QQ was furious with his current therapist, as well as with his prior clinician, for what he experienced as "putting me through torture" in their sessions. That is, rather than experiencing the sessions as relieving his depression, Mr. QQ experienced them as hurtful and harmful. These feelings were particularly strong when the therapist was inquiring about Mr. QQ's painful family conflicts. Many sessions passed in which the patient complained not only that therapy was not helping him but also that it was actually making his depression worse. Transference interpretations in which the therapist pointed out how often Mr. QQ expected him to behave like his mother and siblings were experienced as unhelpful.

The therapist, deeply concerned about the precarious state of the therapeutic alliance, decided to discuss with his patient how the sessions could become more helpful:

> THERAPIST: What might we be able to do to make the sessions less painful for you?
>
> MR. QQ: I think that sometimes you're just too pushy. You want me to talk about all these painful issues all the time, and I just don't feel like doing it. It just makes me feel worse.
>
> THERAPIST: You mean that you would feel like talking about it sometimes but not as often as we do?
>
> MR. QQ: Yes. It's just too much for me.
>
> THERAPIST: It sounds like you would like to have more control over how much we pursue things.
>
> MR. QQ: Yes. I feel like I'm just vulnerable and you keep attacking me.
>
> THERAPIST: That sounds a lot like your descriptions of your mother with you.
>
> MR. QQ: Yes. I guess it does feel like that. But I also think it would really help if you let me decide how much we could talk about certain topics. This stuff about my family is just too hard.
>
> THERAPIST: I think that we should try that, then. I'm sorry if you felt that I wasn't responding to your need to stop stirring up all the painful feelings.

The patient had been experiencing the therapist's probes as having the intrusive quality of the abusive, critical behavior he had experienced with his mother. He felt that he was vulnerable and had no control over the content of the sessions, and he experienced the vulnerability in an increasingly angry and paranoid manner. This led to an enactment in which the frustrated therapist would only press harder to get the patient to pursue more painful topics. Patient and therapist would dig in their heels, leading to a stalemate. After this discussion, the therapist shifted his stance, allowing the patient to signal him when the discussion was becoming too uncomfortable. Although the therapist was initially concerned that avoiding more difficult topics and feelings would lead to an unproductive treatment, he found that Mr. QQ and he made more progress through this approach. The patient did steadily pursue painful topics over the course of the ensuing sessions when he felt that he could do this at his own pace.

Patients With More Severe Narcissistic Sensitivity

Although depressed patients frequently have narcissistic sensitivity, in some cases patients have particularly severe forms, bordering on paranoia. Such severe forms may be an aspect of a comorbid narcissistic or borderline personality disorder (see Chapter 12). These patients may interpret benign statements as negative or have a gift for finding a potential criticism or rejection in a statement meant to be helpful. If their sensitivity is severe enough, they may benefit from atypical antipsychotic agents if these feelings have not resolved with the use of antidepressants.

From the therapeutic standpoint, therapists can reassure these patients that they did not intend to be rejecting or hurtful, and that it is important to understand why the patients heard the comment in this way. Although these patients may not believe their therapists, examination of recurrent instances over time can help them explore the possibility that they are interpreting their therapists' comments in a negative manner that was not intended. Genetic interpretations, along with the transference interpretations, are frequently of value, as many of these patients have experienced traumatic or disrupted developmental histories.

Case Example 2

Ms. RR, a 42-year-old administrative assistant who had repeated severe depressive episodes, experienced almost ceaseless criticism and disparagement from her mother in childhood and as an adult about her appearance, intelligence, weight, and personality. She described her father as either uninterested or not doing anything to actively intervene with her mother, and also as inappropriately touching her.

In this session, Ms. RR brought up her rather characteristic feelings of rejection by the therapist:

> Ms. RR: At the end of last session, you said, "I'll see you on Thursday." You seemed happy to have session over with. You were saying, *I don't want to see you until Thursday.*

THERAPIST: Well, it was certainly not my intention to convey that. In fact, I think I often say that at the end of the session.

MS. RR: Maybe you do, but it felt different this time. I know all I did was complain the last session.

THERAPIST: I know you've mentioned that complaining in your family was treated very negatively. Do you think it's possible that you just felt I was going to be critical since you felt you were complaining?

MS. RR: Well, I don't think so. But I'll think about it. I know if I ever complained to my mother, she was furious. Sometimes, she wouldn't talk to me for days.

Although Ms. RR never fully gave up her suspiciousness, over time she felt less rejected by the therapist. This generalized to other areas; she could consider that she was seeing others as rejecting when they actually made benign comments. This had the impact of a significant increase in self-esteem and easing of her depression.

Patients With Severe Trauma

Many patients with depression have a history of trauma, and some have a history of more severe abuse or neglect. A history of severe trauma can contribute to the various difficulties discussed in this chapter, such as impairments in basic trust, severe narcissistic sensitivity, and acting out. These patients may develop an independent posttraumatic stress disorder, or the depressive symptoms may overlap with symptoms of that disorder. They may find it particularly painful and disruptive to explore their traumatic episodes and may at times experience therapy as more disruptive than helpful. Therapists must use patience, empathy, and tact in exploring the trauma over what may be a period of months or years. They must also be alert to countertransference wishes to avoid the painful material.

Case Example 3

Ms. SS, a 25-year-old graduate student, presented with very severe depressive symptoms that were not relieved by a series of medication trials. Ultimately, she experienced partial relief from a monoamine oxidase inhibitor. Ms. SS was preoccupied with the death of her mother by suicide 8 years earlier. She struggled with intense and overwhelming rage at her mother, with severe guilt about her rage. An only child living alone with her mother, she felt that she should have been able to prevent the suicide. She also experienced a tremendous sense of hopelessness and despair about her life. In fact,

Ms. SS had withdrawn from many aspects of her life, other than her ongoing employment. When the therapist attempted to explore her feelings about her mother's death, Ms. SS would either become deeply despairing and suicidal or refuse to talk, saying that it was pointless. The therapist frequently wondered whether therapy was anything other than painful torture for the patient. Consultants also remained puzzled about what to do.

After about a year into treatment, Ms. SS revealed that she had kept a diary of the events that occurred during her adolescence. The therapist asked her if she would bring it in. Over a few sessions, Ms. SS presented data from her journal. It included painful recollections of the mother's level of depression and rejecting behavior toward the patient. However, there were also positive periods. Unexpectedly, there was a particularly positive discussion with the mother just a few days before her suicide. This helped Ms. SS to realize that she really could not have anticipated the suicide or have known to do more at that time to help her mother. The relief she felt from this discovery helped her to turn a corner in her life and in therapy. For the first time, she seemed to consider the possibility that she could have a life of her own beyond her mother's death.

As noted in this case example, therapists frequently obtain a consultation in the case of patients with severe and persistent depressive disorders. Consultants can review medication treatments that have been employed and assess whether something in the psychotherapeutic approach or countertransference may be contributing to the persistent symptoms. Therapists need not be concerned that patients will see this as an admission of incompetence, as patients typically appreciate therapists' efforts to double-check their work and bring another viewpoint to the situation. If patients do experience the referral for consultation as an admission of uncertainty or as a possible rejection (an attempt to "get rid of" them), this can be explored and may even be helpful in allowing examination of previously overlooked aspects of the transference.

The Negative Therapeutic Reaction

Freud identified a group of patients who had an adverse reaction to treatment when their symptoms began to improve (Freud 1923). He described this phenomenon as a *negative therapeutic reaction* and attributed it to guilty reactions patients had to becoming victors in the oedipal struggle. Success and improvement meant that they were unconsciously succeeding in defeating the same-sex parent while winning over the other. Such a victory might trigger intense guilt and the need to punish themselves by undermining their success or disrupting analytic treatment. More broadly, guilty feelings about success, assertion, and improvement should be explored to prevent a disruption in the therapeutic process.

Case Example 4

Mr. TT was a 46-year-old lawyer who entered psychotherapy with a major depression. Mr. TT described a difficult childhood relationship with his father, who was highly critical and made intellectual demands on the patient that he could not possibly meet. His struggle was complicated by the fact that his father was a very successful entrepreneur who was highly regarded by the community. When Mr. TT was 12 years old, his father died suddenly after a heart attack. Mr. TT felt relieved by his father's death and reported that his life actually improved after that. However, he developed an underlying guilt about his assertiveness and competitiveness, coupled with a fantasy that he had somehow killed his father.

On entering therapy, Mr. TT denied significant conflict about his father's death and reported little in the way of guilty feelings. Therapist and patient became aware, however, of a pattern in which Mr. TT behaved self-destructively as his success at work increased. He would enter into conflicts with superiors or make errors on important documents. Such self-destructive behavior would also occur when Mr. TT made important progress in therapy. After particularly productive periods in his treatment, he would start to come very late to therapy sessions, diluting their impact.

> THERAPIST: I wonder how we can understand your lateness here, and also all the troubles you're starting to have at work again. You had been doing so well until this point!
>
> MR. TT: Well, I agree with what you've pointed out. This kind of setback does seem to come after successes. I guess I agree that it seems as if I'm punishing myself for something.
>
> THERAPIST: I know you felt as if you were better off when your father died. But I think you may feel guilty about that—that sense of relief—without even realizing it.
>
> MR. TT: Well, I guess so. You know, I remember that he seemed to attack me most when I learned new things or wanted to show off my knowledge to him. He would say I was stupid and a know-nothing.
>
> THERAPIST: It sounds like you felt he couldn't tolerate your being successful.
>
> MR. TT: Yes, and I guess for the first time, I'm getting angry about it. I mainly felt frightened before.

Over time, the identification of this pattern helped Mr. TT to become more comfortable with success and with the positive effects of the therapy and diminished negative therapeutic reactions.

Asch (1976) described other dynamics that may be involved in a negative therapeutic reaction. These included patients' identification with a parent who was a suffering martyr. These patients would incorporate this behavior as an ego ideal and feel a loss of the relationship to the parent if they became successful rather than suffering. He also described a group of patients who do not want to accept what the therapist offers because they experience the acceptance as a frightening passive submission.

Difficulty Tolerating the Therapeutic Situation With Increased Acting Out

Some patients who have difficulty with feelings and fantasies that are emerging in the therapeutic situation may increase acting-out behaviors (i.e., risky, aggressive, and self-destructive actions) rather than experience and verbalize painful feelings that are difficult to tolerate. The acting out can derive from emotions and somatic states that cannot be represented and contained symbolically and can also function as a defense against painful feelings and fantasies (Busch and Sandberg 2014). The behaviors may symbolically express the content of what is being warded off. The task of the therapist is to explore the sources and meanings of the behavior and help patients identify the threatening painful feelings and fantasies triggering the acting out. Therapists should encourage patients to avoid risky behavior and to note the feelings and fantasies they have preceding it. If such behavior worsens, a consultation is in order, and the patient may even require a hopefully temporary respite from therapy.

In terms of sources of acting-out behavior, Asch (1976) noted one therapeutic situation in which patients experience themselves as tortured by a sadistic analyst. These patients may not be able to step back and examine this as a transference fantasy or may even provoke analysts into behaving sadistically. Such patients may increase self-destructive behaviors as an expression of their rage, fear, and struggle with therapists. Therapists must monitor their countertransference in reaction to such behaviors and work to help patients understand that their perception of the analyst is actually based on a transference fantasy.

Case Example 5

Mr. UU, a 48-year-old accountant, married with no children, had significant difficulty tolerating his depressive feelings. Whenever they were stirred up in a session, he would invariably go out that night to a bar and drink too much. He would pick up a woman and have a brief sexual encounter, return home to his suspicious and upset wife, and then feel intensely guilty. At times, this made him question whether he could really tolerate therapy. His usual tendency was to repress and deny depressed feelings and avoid situations that might cause them. Mr. UU began to experience the therapy as possibly too upsetting and as posing a potential risk to his marriage.

Various interventions were attempted, in addition to interpretive exploration of the patient's fantasies about the sexual behaviors and about his depressed feelings. Mr. UU was convinced he did not have alcoholism, as he had historically only one or two weekend binges a year, arranged around work holidays, tolerated by his wife, and seen as not disrupting his career or his relationships. Nevertheless, the therapist suggested a consultation with an addiction specialist, whose expertise included finding ways to help people tolerate difficult feelings without drinking, such as using massages, meditation, and yoga. The therapist also added a mood stabilizer to the patient's antidepressant regimen. These interventions were modestly helpful.

However, ongoing exploration as to why feeling depressed was so intolerable ultimately bore fruit. It emerged that Mr. UU had a painful identification with both his mother's and his grandmother's depressions that he had witnessed as a child. He felt vulnerable, sad, and confused when these important nurturers were depressed and unavailable, but his father and brother teased him about these sad feelings. Being depressed came to mean being a target, pathetic, and unmanly. Mr. UU feared that his passivity and sadness meant he might be gay, and he had to frantically reassure himself of his masculinity. But the acting out, although aimed unconsciously at undoing this sense of himself as impaired and damaged, actually contributed to making him feel more unmanly: as a bad husband who might be rejected by his wife. Once Mr. UU understood these previously unconscious fears and their unrealistic nature, his destructive behaviors gradually disappeared.

Although patients with persistent depression sometimes frustrate or overwhelm their therapist with apparently unremitting symptoms and negative therapeutic attitudes, they often slowly respond to consistent and patient exploration of the sources of their symptoms and attention to the transference and therapeutic alliance. As described in this chapter, multiple factors can contribute to their prolonged depressions, and identifying and addressing each of the relevant psychological configurations is of value. Such patients usually require a longer-term psychotherapeutic intervention as well as frequent assessment by the therapist of countertransference reactions.

References

Asch SS: Varieties of negative therapeutic reaction and problems of technique. J Am Psychoanal Assoc 24(2):383–407, 1976 932408

Busch FN, Sandberg LS: Unmentalized aspects of panic and anxiety disorders. Psychodyn Psychiatry 42(2):175–195, 2014 24828589

Freud S: The ego and the id (1923), in The Standard Edition of the Complete Psychological Works of Sigmund Freud, Vol 19. Translated and edited by Strachey J. London, Hogarth Press, 1961, pp 6–63

14

Psychodynamic Approaches to Suicidality

SUICIDE is a significant potential risk in patients with depressive disorders. In this chapter, we describe how psychodynamic psychotherapy can aid in understanding and alleviating the psychological sources of suicidal thoughts. Although an understanding of dynamics is helpful in management of suicidality, we do not focus on management issues. Initial efforts with suicidal patients should focus on ensuring their safety by way of appropriate evaluation of any suicidal ideas or behavior, possible use of medication, and consideration of the need for hospitalization. For further discussion of these practical management issues, we recommend Blumenthal and Kupfer (1990) and Ellison (2001). In some instances, practical management issues supersede psychodynamic exploration. Nevertheless, where possible, the clinician can maintain the inquiring stance consistent with psychodynamic treatment or explore psychodynamic factors alongside implementing practical interventions.

The psychodynamic psychotherapist focuses on the precipitants and meanings of suicidal ideation and behavior. For example, in the case of Ms. SS, described below in Case Example 2, the fantasies about taking an overdose represented an important basis of identification and connection with her mother. As with depression, several dynamic etiologies of suicidality have been described. Kaslow et al. (1998) observed four core overlapping concepts in the psychoanalytic understanding of suicide: the self-directed aggression described by Freud (1917), a pathological grief reaction to the death of an important figure in the patient's life, poor ego functioning with an impairment of reality testing, and pathological representations of self and others. In accord with Freud's theories of depression, Kaslow et al. (1998) viewed suicide as representing murderous feelings toward an ambivalently held other that are turned toward the self when it is identified with that rejecting, disappointing, or lost other. Freud (1917) stated that "no neurotic harbours thoughts of suicide which he has not turned back upon himself from murderous impulses against others..." (p. 252). In this view, suicide corresponds to the dynamics already elaborated in this text for depression, but with an extreme shift toward the enactment of fantasies of self-directed rage.

Pathological grief can manifest as an inability to tolerate, accept, or mourn the loss of a significant other and can culminate in powerful fantasies of reuniting with a lost person through death (Asch 1980; Fenichel 1945). Ego deficits that may increase the risk of suicide include impaired reality testing, often in the context of regression, and the inability to integrate aspects of the self, particularly more positive self-views with the intensely negative self-perceptions that occur in depression. In object relations theory, suicidal patients are viewed as having hostile internal representations of themselves and others, with few positive, soothing self and other representations. The suicidal individual attempts in fantasy to destroy those parts of the self seen as unwanted or bad. According to Asch (1980), ridding oneself of the objectionable parts of the self can represent a symbolic cleansing, allowing one to again be loved by a significant other.

Patients at risk for suicide can also experience themselves as victims of a tormenting other. Asch (1980) described how suicidal individuals may experience the tormenting other as a fantasized executioner. They may attempt to provoke others into attacking them, which then increases their sense of worthlessness and suicidality. One function of this fantasy or behavior is to avert painful feelings of guilt toward the significant other for aggressive or murderous wishes, as these individuals see the aggression as outside themselves. In addition, in viewing themselves as victims, these patients reestablish a relationship with the lost other, although they experience the relationship as one with a torturer rather than with a person they trust.

In addition to the factors described above, patients can experience suicide as revenge against a rejecting other (Menninger 1933) as a means of protecting the rejecting other from the patients' aggression, and as a guilty self-punishment for aggressive and murderous fantasies. Often, patients' suicidal fantasies and behaviors represent a complex admixture of the dynamics described above. Therefore, the clinician may have to illuminate and explore a variety of dynamics. Each of the following cases highlights a specific central dynamic of the patient's suicidality, but it is also clear that other dynamics described in this introduction are also present.

Suicide as Revenge

Although suicide is typically viewed as a murderous hatred expressed toward the self, patients often have more conscious fantasies of revenge against the person or people they see as rejecting. Although openly stated suicidal thoughts and behaviors are important signals of suicide risk, they can also be an expression of vengeful or aggressive wishes toward others.

Case Example 1A

Mr. VV, a 40-year-old businessman, was significantly frustrated with his life, feeling dissatisfied with both his marriage and his career. He felt inadequate at his job and unable to achieve the brilliant work successes he craved. In addition to his current depression, Mr. VV had lifelong dysthymia and was chronically convinced that he was disregarded by others because of his lackluster achievements. Mr. VV longed for fame and attention but had been thwarted in previous attempts at high-profile careers, such as acting. He found his current work pedestrian and unappealing.

Mr. VV had felt chronically neglected and criticized by his parents, contributing to his relentless quest for attention and ongoing sense of failure. His mother had been quite distracted by the chronic, severe illness of a younger sibling, toward whom Mr. VV felt competitive and guilty. His father demanded high levels of achievement from his children, and Mr. VV felt pressured to "make up" for his younger brother's disability. Any expression by Mr. VV of anger at his parents was followed by a strong reprimand, leaving him feeling humiliated and guilty. Mr. VV's older brother, in contrast, seemed to "fit the bill" of his father's needs, demonstrating a consistently high level of academic and athletic achievement. Mr. VV's fantasies of stardom and brief pursuit of an acting career were an attempt to heal his intense feelings of inadequacy but also to rebel against the father's strict standards of appropriate business-oriented professions, to which he nonetheless ultimately drifted.

In the context of ongoing psychotherapy that had helped identify some of the contributions to his dysthymia, Mr. VV experienced an exacerbation of his depression when he failed to obtain an important promotion at work. Although he would have another opportunity for promotion in 2 years, Mr. VV felt that he had fulfilled his father's pronouncements about his inadequacy. He began voicing suicidal thoughts of taking an antidepressant overdose or of shooting himself with a gun. He also voiced anger toward his therapist for "failing him." The therapist explored these feelings with Mr. VV:

> MR. VV: I think that you must have done a bad job if I'm feeling like this now. I think you should be suffering, too.
>
> THERAPIST: You're very disappointed and angry with me. Do you feel like this when you're having the suicidal thoughts?
>
> MR. VV: Yes. I feel that if I killed myself, I'd get my revenge on my parents and on you. I think you would feel like a failure, like you had let me down.
>
> THERAPIST: That sounds a lot like how you feel with your father. You would want me to feel a similar way?
>
> MR. VV: I guess so, although that's not what I had in mind. I also think you'll remember me then. You'll feel badly about your failure with me.
>
> THERAPIST: It sounds like you'll not only get revenge on me, and thereby on your father, but also make a big impact on me.
>
> MR. VV: Yes. I guess so. I never thought I could make much of an impression on people, sandwiched as I was between my brothers. I guess I've always felt extremely angry about that.

As can be seen from this vignette, although revenge was an important factor in the patient's suicidal fantasies, a complex web of dynamics emerged. The patient wished to destroy himself for his failure: he did not feel he deserved to live, demonstrating a severe superego that echoed his father's harsh criticisms. In addition, he wished to punish the parent-analyst for failing him by forcing him to experience the same tormenting worthlessness. Finally, the patient was convinced that this was his only means of creating an impact on the parent-analyst; in a sense, he felt that only through his suicide could he become an important part of the therapist's mind. In fact, the patient admitted fantasizing that the therapist would think about him for many years, trying to understand why he had failed. Exploring these fantasies, especially in the context of the transference, greatly diminished the suicidal thoughts and the pressing depressive symptoms.

Suicide as Pathological Mourning and Wish for Reunion

As described earlier, suicidal fantasies and behavior can be a patient's reaction to the inability to tolerate the loss of an important person. Feelings of rage toward the lost person, guilt, intolerable emptiness or sadness, and wishes for reunion can combine to create the potential for violent behavior toward the self.

Case Example 2

Ms. SS, the graduate student described in Chapter 13, "Managing Impasses and Negative Reactions to Treatment" (see Case Example 3), struggled with severe recurrent depressions. She was often preoccupied with the suicide of her mother 8 years earlier by a medication overdose. Although Ms. SS viewed her mother overall as a chronically angry, depressed, and critical woman, she could sadly recall brief periods when her mother had been lively and fun. This was contrasted with her father, who was extremely involved with his career as an executive at an advertising agency. He worked long hours and was rarely available. Her parents fought constantly when she was present, with her mother regularly attacking her father for his inattentiveness, a complaint that Ms. SS fervently shared. Her parents divorced when she was 14, and the patient was furious with her father for his lack of concern and empathy when her mother died 3 years later.

Ms. SS felt abandoned, enraged with her mother, and preoccupied with a wish to somehow reconnect to her. She focused sadly on her few memories of their positive times together. During the course of therapy, it emerged that for Ms. SS, remaining depressed was a means of staying connected with her mother. She was terrified that should she feel better and go on with her life, she would "lose her mother forever." Ms. SS also struggled with recurrent suicidal thoughts.

> THERAPIST: What kinds of thoughts are you having?
> Ms. SS: I've been thinking about taking all my pills.
> THERAPIST: The same as your mother.
> Ms. SS: Yes. It's true. I've been missing her more recently. If I could only have a chance to spend more time with her! I feel she was mad at me about something, but I'm not sure what. I just feel I was a burden to her.
> THERAPIST: Do you ever have the fantasy that you would join your mother in death?
> Ms. SS: Yes. I do have that fantasy. I'm not a religious person, but sometimes I think that if I died, I would see her again. I just miss her so much.
> THERAPIST: But you are also terribly angry with her.
> Ms. SS: Yeah. I just can't believe she did that to us. How could someone be that unfeeling that they would abandon a child? Sometimes I feel I would also be showing her that she ruined my life.

THERAPIST: I think it's tremendously important that you discover ways of feeling close to your mother or to continue mourning her that don't involve such harm to yourself.

Ms. SS: Well, I do have a lot of diaries that contain memories from that time. I could look through them. But I think it's pretty hopeless. I'm so damaged by what happened.

As noted in Chapter 13, Ms. SS went on to review the extensive diaries from her teens. Revisiting the painful and also the more positive experiences allowed her to work on her anger and feelings of abandonment to a degree. The sense that they had a positive understanding just before her mother suicided and the feeling of reconnecting with her via the diaries relieved some of her own suicidal fantasies and guilt.

Suicide as a Reaction to Experiencing the Other as Torturer

As noted above, the experience of oneself as victim of a tormenting other can be an important factor in suicidal ideation and behavior. The torturer may be internalized as a severely critical superego or experienced, often with some projection, as a significant other in the patient's life. These perceptions of self and others may be based in early traumatic developmental experiences, sometimes with abusive parents. The following cases demonstrate this dynamic—and the value of directly exploring the various meanings of a specific suicidal plan.

Case Example 3

Ms. WW was a 35-year-old single writer who presented for treatment with both dysthymia and several episodes of major depression. She was feeling devastated and lonely after discovering that a man whom she had been seeing on and off for a year was actually living with another woman. Her profession was an isolating one, and she spent a good deal of time alone, though she had one very close female friend.

Ms. WW's family life had been traumatic. She was the third of four siblings, all born fairly close together, to her mother, a Holocaust survivor. Her parents divorced when she was 10, after years of very frightening, dramatic fights that consisted of screaming, pushing, and shoving, often in front of the children. Her mother had a short fuse and would fly into rages and beat the children. Ms. WW had an eating disorder as an adolescent.

Ms. WW began psychoanalysis with sessions four times a week for a low fee. After 7 months, she was addressing considerable transference issues.

She had begun to pay very little and be very late for her sessions, jeopardizing treatment. Discussions about the meaning of these behaviors focused on her "birdlike" eating habits in her teens: she was feeding the therapist little, frustrating amounts, just enough to barely keep the analysis alive, echoing her own intense frustration with what she felt her mother had to offer her, and also in identification with familial Holocaust victims.

Early in the analysis, Ms. WW resumed a relationship with her old boyfriend, even though he continued to live with the other woman. She was furious with him for offering so little (again, like her mother and also in a different way like her father, who had limited contact with her after the divorce) and perceived herself as his victim. She had little ability to see her own aggression—toward herself by remaining in this involvement or toward him in their sadomasochistically tinged sexual encounters. The therapist was beginning to address Ms. WW's aggression in the transference, passively expressed by her refusal to pay her fee, when the boyfriend rejected her. The patient was devastated, ashamed to show her therapist how badly depressed she was, and angry about the therapist's initial interpretations about her aggression. She left her session, just before a 3-day weekend, in a storm, threatening to "maybe" see the therapist for their next appointment.

The therapist heard this as a suicidal threat and decided to call Ms. WW to determine whether that interpretation was correct. In these circumstances of potential suicidality, a call to the patient can be a valuable intervention for assessment and expressing concern for the patient's well-being. Efforts to induce or test the therapist's concern, if present, could be addressed subsequently (see section "Countertransference With Suicidal Patients" later in this chapter). Ms. WW admitted that she had contemplated suffocating herself with a dry-cleaning bag. Exploring the meaning of her suicidal thoughts—first on the phone, then in the next session—therapist and patient learned several important meanings of this fantasy. She was very angry with her therapist and intended in part to express this anger via suicide. She felt that the therapist was "forcing her" to reveal her sexual and aggressive secrets, exposing all of her shameful inadequacies and making her dependent on the treatment—all as a prelude to dropping her from therapy because she was inadequate and not paying the fee. In addition, Ms. WW felt that the therapist, by focusing on her aggression, was being like her mother and older brother, whom she experienced as always telling her how angry and bad she was. She had had many physical fights with her brother, in which he would wrestle her down to the floor and tell her to cry uncle. In one of these fights, he tried to choke her. When she cried or complained, her mother would scream at her for being hysterical, and she would feel that she had to choke back her tears. Now with her therapist, she felt ashamed of her depression and her problems with money and felt that she had to choke back all of it. The idea of suffocating herself related directly to this choking. It was as if she were saying to her mother, brother, and therapist: "Okay, I'll do it! I'll get rid of myself! I'll choke myself to death, so you don't have to do it for me!" Finally, there were obvious gas-chamber references that were not explored in depth, as Ms. WW could not relate to them at the time.

Ms. WW felt very relieved at putting all of this into words and at understanding the multiple specific meanings of her suicidal thoughts. The exploration helped the patient to begin to recognize her own aggression rather than seeing herself simply as the victim of a torturing other. In addition, the ability to reveal these intensely painful feelings reduced her sense of shame and exposure, as the therapist's response was nonjudgmental and helpful.

Case Example 4

Ms. XX, a chemist in her early 30s, began psychotherapy after making a suicide attempt by overdosing on tricyclics. Shortly after starting treatment, she became sharply despondent over a perceived rejection by coworkers. She had learned of some gossip about herself at work, largely about her competitive and aggressive behavior. Ms. XX called her therapist after sitting alone in her apartment for hours, thinking of hanging herself with a belt.

Therapist and patient explored the fantasy in an emergency session. Ms. XX's father had beaten her often with a belt, saying that she was bad for defying his orders, which were usually quite out of touch with her age and social environment. Further, she had often been mocked in school by her peers and called "contaminated," partly because other children found her too aggressive. She was a show-off who liked to call attention to herself, often because she felt bullied and neglected at home. Her mother was ineffective at preventing her father from beating her and knew nothing of her situation with her peers because the patient was too ashamed to confide in her about it.

Learning about the gossip triggered an intense response in which Ms. XX felt hopeless: doomed to be attacked (as by her father and children in past) because she was aggressive and bad, at the same time feeling that it was all untrue and unfair. She turned her rage toward her father and coworkers in the fantasy that she would hang herself with the belt rather than let them hurt her so badly. In addition, she was afraid that her therapist would not be able to help her, just as her mother could not. As she had with her mother, she felt too ashamed and frightened to tell her therapist about this feeling.

Ms. XX's understanding that her suicidal thoughts expressed rage about being attacked helped diminish them dramatically. Speaking about these issues brought enormous relief as well, because she expected to be punished for the rageful thoughts and feelings and was relieved to have them understood and accepted instead.

Suicide as Self-Punishment and Protection of the Other Against Aggression

Suicide frequently represents aggression against a significant rejecting other, turned toward the self. The process by which this occurs may involve complex psychological determinants. It often involves punishment of the self for murderous wishes and may even represent an effort to protect a significant other from murderous fantasies or acts.

Case Example 5

Ms. YY, a 35-year-old secretary, had a long-standing history of aggressive verbal fights with her mother. Generally, Ms. YY felt that she lost these fights. Her mother was extremely critical and seemed to take every opportunity to emphasize her failures. A major focus was on Ms. YY's weight, and her mother blamed her mild obesity for her difficulty keeping a boyfriend.

Ms. YY was troubled by consciously murderous feelings toward her mother, with wishes to be rid of her by any means possible. She vividly imagined battering her until her mother stopped yelling. These fantasies created intense guilt, followed by self-destructive urges.

> THERAPIST: What do you think about the timing of your fantasies, just after you thought of attacking your mother?
>
> Ms. YY: Well, I get frightened that I'm going to hurt her.
>
> THERAPIST: Is it possible that you may think of killing yourself to avoid injuring her?
>
> Ms. YY: Yes, but I don't think it's just that. I also feel suicidal after some of our screaming matches. I just feel very guilty about how I behave, and I have the idea that I'm so bad that I don't even deserve to live.
>
> THERAPIST: What about her attacks toward you?
>
> Ms. YY: That's part of the problem. When I scream at her, I know how much it can hurt. I feel bad that I've behaved the way she did to me.

Ms. YY's dynamics also correspond to those delineated by object relations theorists. She would kill the "bad" aspects of herself, which were identified with her mother's rageful attacks. As Asch (1980) described, Ms. YY unconsciously felt that she would be "purified" by the self-destructive act, allowing her to then be loved by others rather than rejected by her mother, by men, and by certain peers. In addition, Ms. YY's suicidal fantasies included protecting her mother by destroying herself. Her dynamics also suggest identification with the aggressor (see Chapter 10, "Defense Mechanisms in Depressed Patients"), in which the patient feels in the empowered position of the aggressor-mother but then experiences terrible guilt about behaving like her mother.

Suicide as a Function of Impaired Reality Testing and Ego Integration

Suicidal fantasies and behaviors may accompany an impairment in reality testing or a lack of ego integration, particularly in the context of a patient with borderline personality disorder (see Chapter 12, "Psychodynamic Approaches to Depression With Comorbid Personality Disorder"). The patient's defenses are ineffective in managing the intense rage and grieving that triggers these thoughts and behaviors, leaving the feelings unintegrated with the rest of the patient's experience. Impairments in reality testing and ego integrative capacity may also be evidenced by a profound inability to recognize positive aspects of the self, with a focus on the self as worthless and defective.

Case Example 6

Ms. ZZ, a brilliant, attractive, and highly talented musician in her late 20s, made a significant suicide attempt after being rejected by a new boyfriend when he discovered on their third date that she had herpes. Much more prominent than her rage at him and those he represented (especially a distant father) was an intense self-perception of being damaged. Ms. ZZ felt impaired and defective because of the herpes, because of her depression, and because of other deep hurts in the context of her early family life. She felt chronically vulnerable and uncertain about herself because of an entrenched perception of having been the "mousy, unappealing one" in a family of four popular, athletic siblings. Ms. ZZ had never felt able to capture the attention of her socially striving mother or preoccupied, driven father. In this context, her talents had been a source of comfort and even of power to her, though they were not securely integrated into her self-image. Her suicide attempt represented an effort to "wipe herself out" because of the overwhelming fantasy of damage and an absence of ego integration: she could not access any awareness of her significant talents during that suicidal period, viewing herself as "all bad."

It is worth noting that patients with significant depression may have difficulty accessing positive aspects of themselves. Whereas cognitive-behavioral therapy would address evidence that patients view themselves inaccurately, the psychodynamic therapist explores dynamics that contribute to a fantasy of badness (e.g., intense guilt about vengeful feelings). In addition, an inability to identify any positive aspects of the self accompanied by suicidality is suggestive of a biologically based depression and should lead to the consideration of medication (see Chapter 15, "Use of Psychodynamic Psychotherapy With Other Treatment Approaches").

Countertransference With Suicidal Patients

Patients with suicidal feelings can unconsciously or consciously wish to elicit intense emotional reactions from therapists and are sometimes successful at doing so. These can include guilt, worry, and sometimes anger at the patient. In some instances, patients fantasize about the therapist acting as victimizer or even executioner, as described above, and a therapist's anger in these circumstances can trigger fear or guilt that they are enacting this role. It is important for therapists to be alert to these countertransference cues as aids to understanding what patients may be experiencing.

Case Example 1B

As noted earlier in Case Example 1A, Mr. VV attempted to elicit many feelings from the therapist in response to his suicide fantasies and threats. It emerged that in addition to extracting revenge on the therapist by detailing his fantasies about a future suicide, Mr. VV wished the therapist to be actively uncomfortable and fearful for his safety. Mr. VV also longed for the therapist to demonstrate concern for him or reassurance that he was special and loved. For several weeks, the patient succeeded in eliciting the therapist's fear for Mr. VV's safety as well as his anger about feeling manipulated by this patient.

THERAPIST: What means have you thought about for suicide?
MR. VV: I'm not going to discuss any plans with you.
THERAPIST: Why would you not tell me?
MR. VV: I want you to be worried. If you worry about me over the next few days in between sessions, it will show that you care about me.

THERAPIST: I wonder why you feel that you need to do something so drastic to elicit my concern?

MR. VV: I don't know. I guess it's my damn family again. I really had to do so much to get any attention at all. One thing that finally worked was injuring myself. A broken arm was most effective in finally getting someone to notice me!

In this vignette, the therapist used his awareness of the patient's elicitation of fear and concern as a means of understanding Mr. VV's desperate search for responsiveness. In addition, the therapist used his understanding of Mr. VV's background to defuse his own anger about the patient's manipulation, so that this anger would not be enacted through passive hostility or by judgmental interpretations on his part. Through these efforts, the therapist learned that Mr. VV had hoarded medication for a future overdose and convinced him to dispose of it. As Mr. VV realized that the therapist was engaged and wanted to understand him emotionally, he became able to find other ways to communicate his longings, distress, and wish for responsiveness.

Case Example 7

Ms. AAA, a 42-year-old gallery owner, frequently described suicidal thoughts and occasionally made superficial cuts on her wrist. She was often critical of her therapist and devalued him in covert and overt ways. She tended to blame him for her depression and compared him unfavorably to a therapist from her past in another city who "understood me better."

The therapist had to closely monitor his resulting anger at this patient to maintain an engaged therapeutic stance. An example of this occurred when Ms. AAA canceled a session to see a movie with a friend. When her therapist was not able to reschedule the session, Ms. AAA had intensified suicidal thoughts, contemplating making deeper cuts than in the past.

MS. AAA: I felt that when you said you didn't have time, you were rejecting me.

THERAPIST: You thought that I had a time available and I was purposefully withholding it from you?

MS. AAA: Yes. I had that thought—that you were mad at me for canceling the session because of a social engagement. And when I called you, I was feeling really awful!

THERAPIST: You know, you didn't mention how bad you were feeling when you called me! It seems almost as if you're intent on experiencing me as hurtful and rejecting. Maybe sometimes you even try to provoke me to get angry, like canceling the session for reasons that you acknowledge were purely social.

MS. AAA: Yes. That's when I got the thought, "Maybe I should kill myself. Even my shrink hates me!"

THERAPIST: At that point, you can't recognize your own role in precipitating this experience of rejection. I wonder what that is all about!

Thus, the therapist used his experience of frustration to recognize the patient's devaluing, undermining behavior. He then could communicate this perception to the patient, helping her to become aware of her provocative behaviors in the transference. Over time, Ms. AAA was able to understand her pattern of experiencing the therapist as a victimizer, connected to early experiences of intense criticisms by her mother about her intelligence and negative comparisons to her academically successful sister. She also began to appreciate the ways in which she actually elicited this behavior from others, out of guilt over her chronically rageful thoughts and to repeat an early relationship that was familiar to her. These recognitions led to a dramatic reduction in her suicidal thoughts and wrist cutting, as she began to recognize them as rageful, hurt responses to people whom she often erroneously viewed as tormenting her.

As these cases demonstrate, suicidal ideation and behavior can have complex psychological origins: They can represent revenge against others, rage at disappointing others directed against the self, experience of the self as tortured or victimized, difficulty grieving a lost other, and/or the presence of impaired reality testing and ego deficits. Exploring the contribution of these various factors can aid patients in understanding misperceptions that trigger self-destructive acts and help them find more effective and productive means of coping with disappointments and rage. Understanding developed from exploration of patients' suicidality can be usefully applied to other aspects of their depressive disorders.

References

Asch SS: Suicide and the hidden executioner. Int Rev Psychoanal 7:51–60, 1980

Blumenthal SJ, Kupfer DJ (eds): Suicide Over the Life Cycle: Risk Factors, Assessment and Treatment of Suicidal Patients. Washington, DC, American Psychiatric Press, 1990

Ellison JM (ed): Treatment of Suicidal Patients in Managed Care. Washington, DC, American Psychiatric Press, 2001

Fenichel O: The Psychoanalytic Theory of Neurosis. New York, WW Norton, 1945

Freud S: Mourning and Melancholia (1917 [1915]), in The Standard Edition of the Complete Psychological Works of Sigmund Freud, Vol 14. Translated and edited by Strachey J London, Hogarth Press, 1957, pp 239–258

Kaslow NJ, Reviere SL, Chance SE, et al: An empirical study of the psychodynamics of suicide. J Am Psychoanal Assoc 46(3):777–796, 1998 9795891

Menninger KA: Psychoanalytic aspects of suicide. Int J Psychoanal 14:376–390, 1933

Use of Psychodynamic Psychotherapy With Other Treatment Approaches

PSYCHODYNAMIC psychotherapy can be integrated fairly readily with other treatments, including medication, cognitive-behavioral therapy (CBT), and couples therapy. Patients treated with psychodynamic therapy for depression frequently also take antidepressant or mood-stabilizing medications for their symptoms, which is sometimes essential for a full exploration of their conflicts. When medication treatments are so complex as to limit time available for psychotherapy, or when the therapist is not a physician, a psychopharmacologist can manage the patient's medications. The use of medication and the therapist's role in employing this modality (whether the therapist or another health professional is prescribing) can often be important areas for exploration. For additional discussion of the issues involved in combining psychodynamic psychotherapy with other treatments, see Beitman and Klerman (1991), Riba and Balon (2001), Kay (2001), and Busch and Sandberg (2007).

Aspects of CBT can also be congruent with psychodynamic psychotherapy. In fact, certain components of depression-focused psychodynamic psychotherapy can be seen as "cognitive," such as clarifying for patients the unrealistic nature of their self-criticisms. However, in CBT these interventions are central, whereas in psychodynamic psychotherapy they are a step toward exploration of the meanings of patients' self-criticism, the dynamic issues and conflicts underlying their symptoms, and the developmental contributors to their illness. In some instances, patients can benefit from being in both treatments simultaneously. For example, in the case of Mr. BBB (discussed below in "Case Example 1"), cognitive-behavioral work on his sexual dysfunction helped him to feel more comfortable exploring this symptom in much greater depth in his psychodynamic treatment, which was crucial for his full recovery from depression.

Psychodynamic Psychotherapy and Medication

Determining Whether to Use Medication With Psychodynamic Psychotherapy

Medication should always be considered for patients with a major depressive disorder. For milder or moderate depressive episodes, therapists can attempt a treatment with therapy alone. Evidence suggests that more severe depressions respond better to medication or combined treatment than to psychotherapy alone (American Psychiatric Association 2010; Elkin et al. 1989). Elements in the decision-making process should include the level of the patient's suffering and the degree to which the depressive symptoms interfere with the patient's functioning and the psychotherapeutic process. Medications should almost always be used if the patient demonstrates a suicide risk. If the patient's symptoms are not responding to psychotherapy alone after 2–3 months, medication should be reconsidered. At each point in the decision-making process, patients should be informed of the risks and benefits of the various interventions so that they can take an appropriate part in planning their treatment. Patients can often participate in making decisions about the use of medication, a form of treatment that Gutheil (1978) called "participant prescribing." In psychodynamic treatment, both the decision and the conflicts that may affect the decision are explored.

Case Example 1

Mr. BBB, a 43-year-old stock analyst, presented with depressive symptoms in the setting of conflicts with his wife. They had not been sexually involved for several years, and he was very frustrated with her. In part, he steered away from sex because he felt that his wife was not passionate, and he was chronically dissatisfied with their rather perfunctory lovemaking. Mr. BBB had been briefly involved with another woman whom he found to be much more passionate but felt very guilty about this. He withdrew emotionally in the relationship, and the woman then ended their affair.

Mr. BBB described significant symptoms of depression, including intense guilty preoccupations, middle and terminal insomnia, and a weight loss of 6 pounds over the prior 2 months. Nevertheless, he could function at his job and denied any suicidality. The therapist recommended the use of medication:

THERAPIST: I think that medication would be very helpful to you.

MR. BBB: I don't think that's really necessary. I'm able to do my work.

THERAPIST: You may be able to function, but you are really suffering from your guilty thoughts and feelings, and you are struggling with your energy, sleep, and weight.

MR. BBB: I think my guilt is understandable. I did betray my wife.

THERAPIST: It's not just the intensity of your guilt that indicates you may have a biochemical problem. It's also the other symptoms you describe.

MR. BBB: Well, if there's any other way to do it, I'd prefer it. I'm really against medication.

THERAPIST: I wonder if your guilt may be playing a role in your decision. I wonder if you're punishing yourself by allowing your depression to persist.

MR. BBB: That sounds right. I think I may be doing other self-punishing things as well that I'd like to talk to you about. Maybe my problem with medication is part of that. Nevertheless, I'd like to try therapy first.

The therapist clearly thought that medication in conjunction with psychotherapy would be most helpful for this patient. Ultimately, the patient decided against it, but the discussion paved the way for further exploration of Mr. BBB's guilt and a strengthening of the therapeutic alliance. Mr. BBB was more willing to consider medication in the future, as the therapeutic alliance became more established and as he understood more about the relationship of his refusal of relief for guilt over the affair. To Mr. BBB, too, it was important that he feel in control of this decision, rather than helpless and pressured by the therapist to accept medication. In instances in which the depressive symptoms may be dangerous, however, it may be necessary to press harder to convince a patient to take antidepressant medication.

Shame About Psychotherapeutic or Psychopharmacological Interventions

As described in prior chapters, patients often experience shame about their depression, and the illness itself tends to exacerbate self-critical tendencies and the feeling of being a bad person. Patients may therefore resist treatments if they experience these interventions as further indications that they are indeed bad or defective, as another narcissistic injury. Thus, they may use medication as a resistance to psychotherapy, if they see the need for therapy as shameful, or they may resist medication if they view this need as a source of shame (Busch and Auchincloss 1995). Addressing these particular resistances can be valuable, particularly when patients would be best served by a combination treatment.

Case Example 2

Mr. CCC, a 58-year-old retired sales executive, entered treatment with severe depression and vegetative symptoms. His depression had begun at about the time he retired, a year earlier. Initial interviews pinpointed multiple stresses. Retirement had not gone particularly well for Mr. CCC. He was bored and tense with his wife, because he was at home with her much of the time. Mr. CCC became irritable and critical of her, and she in turn became increasingly withdrawn. In addition, after a few sessions Mr. CCC shamefully revealed that rather than voluntarily retiring, as he had suggested initially, he had been forced out of his position at his firm when new management took over. He remained quite angry and hurt, although he had difficulty discussing these issues.

Mr. CCC recounted an early history of being quite close to his father. The only son of five children, Mr. CCC experienced himself as his father's favorite. They often had played games and spent enjoyable time in each other's company. However, when he became a teenager, his father not only became more distant but also criticized him as being a "loser" and inept. His recent job loss, accompanied by a sense of being unwanted, was experienced very much like the withdrawal of his father's love, and then, as now, the patient felt inadequate and humiliated.

Mr. CCC readily agreed to medication but was quite resistant to psychotherapy, despite finding the link between his current feelings and early life experience to be of interest. After Mr. CCC's symptoms partially responded to medication, he stated that he no longer needed any therapy and that his improvement showed that his illness was purely "biological." The therapist, however, felt that Mr. CCC had an ongoing susceptibility to feeling inadequate, criticized, and humiliated during his retirement. The therapist explored this with Mr. CCC:

> THERAPIST: I certainly agree that your symptoms have improved on medication, but you still seem unfulfilled by your current lifestyle, frustrated with your wife, and feeling inadequate and upset about your forced retirement. Why do you think you don't want to explore these issues further in psychotherapy?

> MR. CCC: I really think that evidence shows that my depression was a biological problem. I feel somewhat better, and I don't think much more can be done about it.
>
> THERAPIST: What is your specific concern about psychotherapy?
>
> MR. CCC: Well, I think that medications simply mean I have an illness that needs to be treated. When you bring up therapy, it feels as if you are blaming me for what's happening. Like somehow this is my fault.
>
> THERAPIST: It sounds like your father's ridicule of you—as if I am saying that you are a loser.
>
> MR. CCC: Yes. I guess it does. It seems silly to think of it that way, but that's how it feels.

This intervention helped Mr. CCC to engage in a psychotherapeutic process aimed at addressing the difficulties that seemed to contribute to his unhappiness. The example also demonstrates how early interventions that explore the patient's experience of the therapist can pave the way for later transference work. Mr. CCC's transference fantasy of the therapist as a loving father who would eventually, however, withdraw and attack became a core issue in the patient's treatment.

The type of struggle Mr. CCC experienced can frequently occur in the other direction, with the patients experiencing medication as a sign that they are defective. Explorations of various dynamic meanings of medication can be helpful overall in the therapeutic process but may be of particular importance in overcoming resistances to this modality when the therapist feels it is important in treating the depression.

Case Example 3

Ms. DDD, a 25-year-old actress, experienced a recurrence of depression while taking medication. On further inquiry, Ms. DDD revealed that she had not been taking the medication consistently, and the recurrence had occurred in this context. It emerged that Ms. DDD experienced being prescribed medication as a narcissistic injury, another sign that she was defective. She felt that taking antidepressants contributed to her sense of isolation from and jealousy of others, feelings that she had often experienced as a child and adolescent. In contrast to the other children she knew, Ms. DDD had viewed herself as less wealthy and not as cool. In addition, she felt that her father had little interest in her and assumed that this was because she was unappealing and unattractive. Currently, difficulties in succeeding at her acting career, including being rejected for roles, had stimulated these feelings of inadequacy and defectiveness. Such rejections and her emotional reactions to them appeared to generally trigger recurrences of depressive episodes. Thus, early life stresses and negative appraisals of herself in relation to others seemed to trigger a biochemically based depression, which further exacerbated her view of herself as inadequate. Medication had helped to relieve this cycle.

Her therapist found it essential, then, to explore with Ms. DDD her difficulties in complying with treatment with antidepressants:

THERAPIST: I want to try to understand why you weren't taking your medication regularly, particularly given how problematic your depressions are for you.

MS. DDD: I feel that it means I'm defective in some kind of way. How come I have this problem? My friend was able to stop her Prozac after 3 months.

THERAPIST: It's important for us to address your depression individually, and we've found that the medication is very helpful for you. In what way does it make you feel defective?

MS. DDD: Just that something is wrong with me and that other people won't be interested in being with me.

THERAPIST: It sounds a lot like what you've described experiencing for so many years when you were growing up.

MS. DDD: Yes, always feeling ignored or left out. I guess my father is the most painful example. He was always working, and when he came home, all he did was watch TV. I guess I've just always felt something is wrong with me.

THERAPIST: Well, I think it's important to understand more about how the medication became intertwined with these beliefs, especially when it's relieved your depression in the past and when that depression makes you feel so much worse about yourself.

MS. DDD: I guess I should be a lot more careful about it—I really don't want to be so negative about myself all the time. I just feel really angry with my father, and I think I'm envious of my friend who doesn't need her Prozac anymore. Maybe I need to talk more about that.

Medication as an Aid to Psychotherapy

In many cases, depression and its associated symptoms can disrupt the psychotherapeutic exploratory process. Medication may be essential not just to relieve the depressive symptoms but also to allow psychodynamic psychotherapy to proceed.

Case Example 4

Ms. EEE, a 33-year-old interior decorator with a history of recurrent depression and obsessions, presented with persistent fears that her husband was tiring of her and wanted to leave her for another woman. However, her description of him indicated that he was actually devoted to their relationship and had no interest in an extramarital involvement. Ms. EEE felt tormented by these preoccupations, which became so severe that they disrupted her functioning. She could reality-test these ideas at times but could hold on to a realistic perspective for only brief periods.

Attempts to explore the origin of Ms. EEE's symptoms in therapy proved difficult because of the patient's obsessive questioning of the therapist about his view of her husband's attitude and behavior: *Don't men always want to be involved with someone outside the marriage? Don't couples get bored with each other?* Attempting to explore her fears usually exacerbated them, and attempts at reassurance eased this patient's distress for only brief intervals.

Given her clinical picture, Ms. EEE's therapist strongly advised medication. After approximately 2 months of taking a selective serotonin reuptake inhibitor, Ms. EEE experienced a significant reduction in her obsessional preoccupations. Only then could she more fully explore the traumatic impact of early childhood experiences.

This patient's father had been involved in multiple extramarital affairs and regarded her mother with disparagement. To justify his actions, her father would often tell Ms. EEE that couples cannot be expected to remain close to or sexually interested in each other: they are bound to grow apart. Sometimes her father seemed to favor Ms. EEE with special attention that made her feel guilty, as she experienced him as being mean and inattentive to her mother. At other times, however, her father seemed to be uninterested in and critical of the patient. Ms. EEE was very frightened that one day her husband would behave similarly, abandoning her as her father had left her mother when she became older. Medication helped to quell Ms. EEE's obsessional fears and thus allowed her a deeper engagement in psychotherapy. In the context of her diminished anxiety and of the therapeutic focus on her parental relationships, she developed an observing ego with which to reevaluate her current perceptions of her husband.

Psychotherapy as an Aid to Taking Medication

Case Example 5

Ms. FFF was a 30-year-old nurse who presented with chronic depressive symptoms and a long history of intense self-criticism. Despite the significant level of suffering created by her symptoms, Ms. FFF was highly resistant to taking medications. On exploring her resistance, Ms. FFF revealed that she was a child of privilege and did not feel that it was appropriate for her to have problems, because "so many people have real problems and I don't."

The therapist suggested that this viewpoint was connected to general feelings of guilt associated with her depression and stated that it was important to understand these feelings rather than letting them interfere with her getting appropriate treatment. Ms. FFF, however, was still unwilling to proceed, continuing to feel that getting help was an indulgence.

The therapist delved further into Ms. FFF's background to see what might shed light on the origins of her guilty self-deprivation. She reported that her parents were caring but indecisive and inhibited people who also struggled with low self-esteem. Her oldest sister concluded that she needed to be tough on her siblings because her parents were unable to do so. She was highly critical and demanding of the patient, suggesting that many of Ms. FFF's social and academic efforts were inadequate. She would also incite her brothers and father to attack her mother, who seemed to lack common sense in many areas. Ms. FFF felt bad about these attacks and that she had to intervene to protect her mother.

In her treatment, it came to be understood that Ms. FFF saw any emergence of power on her part as potentially damaging to others, just as she saw power misused by her sister. These dynamics suggest the presence of identification with the aggressor (see Chapter 10, "Defense Mechanisms in Depressed Patients"). She reluctantly revealed that she was also quite critical of her mother but felt very guilty about these feelings. Thus, Ms. FFF kept herself in a weakened state with her self-criticisms and her depression. She seemed unaware that she could use her personal power for positive purposes instead of wielding it against others. Helping her realize this possibility aided her in deciding to take medication. As her depression and capabilities gradually improved, the theme of dangerous empowerment had to be revisited repeatedly. In addition, her childhood fear of and anger toward her sister had to be addressed in depth.

Split Treatments: Coordinating Treatments Involving a Psychotherapist and Psychopharmacologist

Much has been written about collaborations of therapists and psychopharmacologists in so-called treatment triangles (Beitman et al. 1984; Busch and Gould 1993; Busch and Sandberg 2007; Kahn 1991; Riba and Balon 2001). There are many ways in which these treatments can go awry or be disrupted, because the relationships are vulnerable to splitting, conflicts over treatment interventions, and professional jealousy. Thus, it is important to maintain productive communication between the two treating clinicians, particularly during treatment difficulties.

Case Example 6

Mr. GGG, a 52-year-old writer, had been successfully treated 3 years earlier for major depression by a psychopharmacologist after referral by his therapist. After approximately 2 years, the patient was doing quite well and his medication was tapered off. However, 1 year later, Mr. GGG's depression recurred when he was competing to be president of an academic organization.

Mr. GGG contacted the psychopharmacologist, who was also a psychoanalyst, and went in for reevaluation. It was clear from the interview that Mr. GGG's depressive symptoms were severe and disrupting his functioning. When the psychopharmacologist recommended medication, Mr. GGG reported that his therapist had expressed wariness about this measure.

> PSYCHOPHARMACOLOGIST: What did he say to you?
>
> MR. GGG: He told me that we understood what was going on, that I was conflicted about competing and was fearful of being too aggressive. He felt the depression was a way of undermining my assertiveness in this situation and avoiding doing damage.
>
> PSYCHOPHARMACOLOGIST: Where did the issue of medication come in, then?
>
> MR. GGG: Well, he said that since we understood this conflict so well, I wouldn't really need the medication. And I certainly agree with what he's saying about my difficulty being competitive, but I'm really suffering. In fact, I feel frustrated that he has not encouraged medications.
>
> PSYCHOPHARMACOLOGIST: Have you spoken to him about this?
>
> MR. GGG: No.
>
> PSYCHOPHARMACOLOGIST: Well, I think it's very important that you bring it up with him, as with any feelings you are having about your therapist. Of course, I'll be speaking with him as well.

When the psychopharmacologist spoke with the therapist, he clarified with the clinician the point that understanding, although often helpful with depression, did not seem in itself to be aiding this particular patient. The therapist agreed that this was the case and felt that he should reevaluate his countertransference, because he was surprised that he had not recognized this earlier. The patient also productively brought up his frustration with the therapist, and they examined it together. Mr. GGG's depressive symptoms resolved within 6 weeks of starting to take the medication, and his therapy remained highly effective.

Psychodynamic Psychotherapy Combined With Other Psychotherapies

Combining Psychodynamic Psychotherapy With Cognitive-Behavioral Therapy

As described above, the techniques of CBT and psychodynamic psychotherapy overlap. Some theoreticians and clinicians have described psychoanalysis as a cognitive and learning treatment in which patients present with certain false and problematic beliefs about themselves, others, and the world. These views have been learned during development in early childhood, and the transference presents an important opportunity for testing these beliefs. Therefore, in addition to pointing out the catastrophic nature of these negative self-perceptions, psychodynamic psychotherapists often address patients' cognitive distortions about the therapist, such as a belief that the therapist is critical of or rejecting them. In CBT, testing and reevaluating cognitions is the central focus of the therapy, but such testing rarely includes beliefs about the therapist. In psychodynamic therapy, the central focus is on exploring the unconscious dynamisms and intrapsychic conflicts that contribute to these cognitive distortions.

Both therapies should be considered in working with depressed patients. Some patients may not be able to work effectively in psychodynamic psychotherapeutic treatment, whereas others may find CBT frustrating or limiting. Patients may work more effectively in one or another form of treatment at various points.

A single therapist will likely face difficulties in attempting to combine the two treatment approaches with one patient. Testing the evidence with regard to cognitions, using homework as a tool, offering prestructured sessions, and avoiding attention to the transference—all characteristic aspects of CBT—often conflict with the more open-ended exploratory stance of the psychodynamic psychotherapist. If the two treatments are employed by separate practitioners, as with a psychoanalyst and psychopharmacologist, it is essential that the treating clinicians collaborate rather than present the patient with competing viewpoints. Ideas that emerge in one or the other treatment can also often be used to supplement material in the other.

Case Example 7

Mr. HHH, a 32-year-old computer technician with recurrent depressive episodes, had severe low self-esteem with regard to women, particularly sexually. To cope with this, he tended to avoid involvement with women, particularly sexual intercourse, in which he was prone to premature ejaculation. Although there was evidence of oedipal conflicts and castration fears, the patient was highly resistant to discussing these fears in therapy, as he found them to be terribly humiliating. Sildenafil was not available at the time of this patient's treatment.

The therapist, a man, referred Mr. HHH to a female sex therapist who specialized in cognitive and behavioral approaches. As Mr. HHH practiced techniques to reduce premature ejaculation and explored these concerns in a more structured, cognitive mode, he began to feel hopeful about dealing with this problem and was more willing to consider the possibility of psychodynamic contributors.

THERAPIST: What do you think helped you to decide to explore this further?

MR. HHH: I found it terribly humiliating before this to talk about sex—it was just too painful. I guess I see some hope now, whereas before it just didn't seem worth the embarrassment.

THERAPIST: Does the sex therapist's being a woman affect things?

MR. HHH: Yes. I felt a lot safer. That made me realize that I was worried about feeling humiliated if I talked to you about it. I guess I was reminded too much of the "dressing-downs" my father would give me when I asked for help about certain things. He just always left me feeling very inadequate.

THERAPIST: And unmanly.

MR. HHH: Yes. That's right. But I feel much more comfortable now speaking with you about it.

Combining Psychodynamic Psychotherapy With Couples Therapy

As with the other treatment approaches described, psychodynamic psychotherapy can be readily integrated with couples treatment. Many couples therapists use psychodynamic techniques in exploring the origins of conflicts within each member of the couple and pay attention to how these may interact to foment discord. Thus, patients can bring the insights gained in couples treatment into their individual psychodynamic therapy for depression, and vice versa. In addition, problems between members of a couple can be an ongoing contributor to stress and to patients' feelings of inadequacy, low self-esteem, and conflicted rage. Easing the conflicts between members of a couple can therefore add to relief of depression.

Case Example 8

Mr. TT, a 46-year-old lawyer discussed in Chapter 13, "Managing Impasses and Negative Reactions to Treatment" (see Case Example 4), had persistent intense feelings of inadequacy and narcissistic vulnerability that were exacerbated by a deteriorating marriage. Mr. TT experienced his wife as viewing him as "toxic," his very presence a source of disgust to her. Thus, Mr. TT would be confined to certain parts of the house to do his work. His wife was critical of him in many areas, particularly about his weaknesses as a father and about his income level. Mr. TT did admit to some difficulties in relating to his children but in no way saw himself as actively damaging them in the manner his wife seemed to suggest.

In part because of his low self-esteem, Mr. TT struggled with questions as to whether his wife was right about the severity of his problems or was instead being malicious or unfair. Some of his perplexity about this issue appeared to develop from confusion in his childhood home about the role of his father. As noted in Chapter 13, his father was a successful entrepreneur who was active in the community and widely admired, including by his mother. However, the patient saw his intensely critical and demanding side. Mr. TT was confused that his father's nastiness went unrecognized and struggled about whether his father was indeed unfair or whether he, himself, was terribly defective. In part to further examine this notion and to see if the marital problems could be reduced, Mr. TT and his wife entered couples therapy.

At first, couples therapy appeared to offer promise. As he felt less depressed, Mr. TT had made many changes, such as participating more in activities with his children, in an attempt to respond to his wife's concerns. However, he found that her criticisms continued. The couples therapist addressed the discrepancy between his changes and her ongoing critiques. His wife responded that the changes thus far were "not enough." In fact, she began to discuss pursuing a divorce.

Mr. TT now felt less confused because he began to realize that no matter what he did, his wife would likely reject him. Further exploration of his father's "hero" status helped clarify the historical determinants for his confusion when faced with others' aggression. Despite this understanding and despite exacerbating tensions that were contributing to a resurgence of his depressive symptoms, Mr. TT was reluctant to end his marriage.

> THERAPIST: Why do you think you don't want a divorce, considering how unhappy your marriage is making you?
> MR. TT: At this point, I really just don't know—I'm so miserable! I feel almost as if I'm punishing myself for something.

THERAPIST: Any ideas what that could be?

In this context, the therapist and patient re-reviewed what they had learned about his experience of his father's sudden death when Mr. TT was 12 years old. His intense guilt about his father's death led to a pattern of recurrent self-destructive and self-punishing behavior.

THERAPIST: Well, I wonder if you are in some ways using the re-lationship with your wife now as a way of keeping yourself down or as punishing yourself for your guilty wishes about your father that seemed to come true.
MR. TT: That may be, because I remember feeling badly that I didn't feel worse. Also, I have noticed that I get worried and guilty when things do go well.

Mr. TT's depression improved greatly shortly after his separation. In this context, his fears and guilt about "things going well" intensified, as did his need to punish himself. These issues became a primary focus of his dynamic treatment. Mr. TT's insights developed in part from the two treatments working together, the couples therapy demonstrating the consensual reality of his wife's aggression and the psychotherapy exploring the reasons for his confusion about her behavior and his tolerating it for so long.

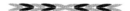

Patients can often benefit from the combination of psychodynamic psy-chotherapy and other types of interventions. As noted previously, we be-lieve that the psychodynamic treatment outlined in this book can reduce symptoms of depression and vulnerability to recurrence of the disorder. Further research will be required, however, to definitively determine which treatment or combinations of treatments are most effective for specific de-pressive disorders or patients. Until such time, it is important to be knowl-edgeable about the broad array of potential interventions and to use clinical judgment, sometimes with the aid of a consultant in more complex cases, in the treatment of depression.

References

American Psychiatric Association: Practice guideline for the treatment of patients with major depressive disorder (third edition). Am J Psychiatry 197(suppl):1–45, 2010

Beitman BD, Klerman GL (eds): Integrating Pharmacotherapy and Psychotherapy. Washington, DC, American Psychiatric Press, 1991

Beitman BD, Chiles J, Carlin A: The pharmacotherapy-psychotherapy triangle: psychiatrist, nonmedical psychotherapist, and patient. J Clin Psychiatry 45(11):458–459, 1984 6490593

Busch FN, Auchincloss EL: The psychology of prescribing and taking medication, in Psychodynamic Concepts in General Psychiatry. Edited by Schwartz HJ, Bleiberg E, Weissman SH. Washington, DC, American Psychiatric Press, 1995, pp 401–416

Busch FN, Gould E: Treatment by a psychotherapist and a psychopharmacologist: transference and countertransference issues. Hosp Community Psychiatry 44(8):772–774, 1993 8375839

Busch FN, Sandberg L: Psychotherapy and Medication: The Challenge of Integration. Hillsdale, NJ, The Analytic Press, 2007

Elkin I, Shea MT, Watkins JT, et al: National Institute of Mental Health Treatment of Depression Collaborative Research Program. General effectiveness of treatments. Arch Gen Psychiatry 46(11):971–982, discussion 983, 1989 2684085

Gutheil TG: Drug therapy: alliance and compliance. Psychosomatics 19(4):219–225, 1978 635081

Kahn DA: Medication consultation and split treatment during psychotherapy. J Am Acad Psychoanal 19(1):84–98, 1991 1676395

Kay J (ed): Integrated Treatment of Psychiatric Disorders (Review of Psychiatry Series; Oldham JM, Riba MB, series eds). Washington, DC, American Psychiatric Publishing, 2001

Riba MB, Balon R (eds): Psychopharmacology and Psychotherapy: A Collaborative Approach. Washington, DC, American Psychiatric Press, 2001

Index

of suicidality as function of
impaired reality testing and
ego integration, 208–209
of suicidality as pathological
mourning and wish for
reunion, 203–204
of suicidality as reaction to experiencing the other as torturer,
204–206
of suicidality as revenge, 201–202
of therapeutic alliance, 48–49
of transference, 149–152
of vulnerability based on perceived difference, 91–92
of whether to use medication with
psychodynamic treatment,
214–215
of working with central themes,
80–81
of working with dreams, 82–83
CBT. *See* Cognitive-behavioral therapy
Central themes, 66
case example of, 80–81
Character
identifying anger, guilt, and self-
punishment in, 131–134
case examples of, 132–134
Chronic persistent depression
(dysthymia), 5, 10, 27. *See also*
Case examples; Depression
Clarification, 66–67
case example of, 66–67
description of, 66
Clomipramine
for treatment of depression, 4
Cognitive-behavioral therapy (CBT),
3, 178
medication and, 222
case example of, 223
Competitiveness
link between aggression and,
111–112
case example of, 111–112

Conflicts
case example of, 77–79
Confrontation, 67–68
case example of, 68
Countertransference
case examples of, 80–81
suicidality with, 209–211
feelings of, 79–81
with negative reactions to treatment, 199
reactions during termination
phase, 168–171
case example of, 168–171
Couples therapy, 223–225. *See also*
Marriage
case example of, 225–226
Cultural norms, 138

DAS (Dysfunctional Attitude Scale),
178
Defense interpretation, 69
Defense Mechanism Rating Scale
(DMRS), 27
Defense mechanisms, 153–162
in depression, 26–27
overview, 153, **154**
against painful affects, **30**
Denial, 154–155
case example of, 154–155
description of, **154**
Depression. *See also* Superego
approaches to depression with
comorbid personality disorder, 175–187
dependent and avoidant personality disorders, 176–177
narcissistic and borderline personality disorders, 179–186
case examples of, 180–186
obsessive-compulsive personality disorder, 177–179
case example of, 178–179
overview, 175–176

CPSIA information can be obtained
at www.ICGtesting.com
Printed in the USA
LVOW04s1001120316

478906LV00003B/4/P